To the nursing students who are our next generation of researchers essential for building an evidence-based practice for nursing.

Susan & Jennifer

In memory of my father Delbert Grove, who was so proud of my publishing activities.

Susan

To my husband, Randy, for supporting my scholarly goals.

Jennifer

We hope that this Study Guide is helpful to you in learning the steps of the research process, critically appraising studies, and synthesizing research findings to facilitate an evidence-based practice for your patients and their families.

Susan K. Grove
Jennifer R. Gray

Reviewers

Jacalyn P. Dougherty, PhD, RN
Nursing Research Consultant
JP Dougherty, LLC
Aurora, Colorado

Joanne T. Ehrmin, RN, COA-CNS, PhD, MSN, BSN
Professor
University of Toledo, College of Nursing
Toledo, Ohio

Tamara Kear, PhD, RN, CNS, CNN
Assistant Professor of Nursing
Villanova University
Villanova, Pennsylvania

Robin Moyers, PhD, RN-BC
Nursing Educator
Carl Vinson VA Medical Center
Dublin, Georgia

Teresa M. O'Neill, PhD, APRN, RNC
Professor
Our Lady of Holy Cross College
New Orleans, Louisiana

Sandra L. Siedlecki, PhD, RN, CNS
Senior Nurse Scientist
Cleveland Clinic
Cleveland, Ohio

Sharon Souter, PhD, RN, CNE
Dean and Professor
University of Mary Hardin Baylor
Belton, Texas

Molly J. Walker, PhD, RN, CNS, CNE
Professor
Angelo State University
San Angelo, Texas

Cindy W. Ward, DNP, RN-BC, CMSRN, ACNS-BC
Surgical Clinical Nurse Specialist
Carilion Roanoke Memorial Hospital
Roanoke, Virginia

Angela F. Wood, PhD, Certified High-Risk Perinatal Nurse
Assistant Professor and Chair
Carson-Newman University, Department of Nursing
Jefferson City, Tennessee

Preface

The amount of knowledge generated through nursing research is rapidly escalating. This empirical knowledge is critical for developing an evidence-based practice in nursing that is both high-quality and cost-effective for patients, families, providers, and healthcare agencies. As a nursing student and registered nurse, you will be encouraged to read, critically appraise, and use research findings to develop protocols, algorithms, and policies for practice. We recognize that learning research terminology and reading and critically appraising research reports are complex and sometimes overwhelming activities. Thus, we have developed this *Study Guide for Understanding Nursing Research* to assist you in clarifying, comprehending, analyzing, synthesizing, and applying the content presented in your textbook, *Understanding Nursing Research*, 6th edition.

The Study Guide is organized into 14 chapters, which are consistent with the chapters of the textbook. Each chapter presents you with learning exercises that require various levels of knowledge and critical thinking skills. These exercises are organized using the following headings: Terms and Definitions, Linking Ideas, Web-Based Information and Resources, and Conducting Critical Appraisals to Build an Evidence-Based Practice. In some exercises, you will define relevant terms or identify key ideas. In other exercises, you will demonstrate comprehension of the research process by linking one idea to another. Another section was developed with exercises to increase your use of web-based resources to locate relevant research information for classroom and clinical activities. In the most complex exercises, you will apply your new research knowledge by conducting critical appraisals of published quantitative and qualitative studies.

This edition of the Study Guide has been revised to include new content relevant for understanding the following steps of the research process: problem, purpose, literature review, framework, ethics, design, sampling, measurement, and statistics. We have expanded and updated the content on qualitative research and included the exploratory-descriptive qualitative research method that is commonly used in nursing studies. The textbook also includes revised and simplified critical appraisal processes for quantitative and qualitative research, and these processes are applied to a current qualitative study and two quantitative studies throughout this Study Guide. The 6th edition of the textbook also includes an extensive expansion of the content on synthesis of research knowledge in building an evidence-based practice. You are provided exercises to facilitate your reading of syntheses of research and using this knowledge in developing evidence-based protocols, algorithms, and policies in clinical agencies.

After completing the exercises for each chapter, you will be able to review the answers in the Answer Key at the back of the book to assess your understanding of the content. Based on your correct and incorrect responses, you will be able to focus your study to improve your knowledge of each chapter's content. We believe that completing the exercises in the Study Guide can provide you with a background for reading, analyzing, and synthesizing the evidence from research reports for application to practice.

HOW TO GET THE MOST OUT OF THIS STUDY GUIDE

The exercises in *Study Guide for Understanding Nursing Research*, 6th edition, were designed to assist you in comprehending the content in your textbook, conducting critical appraisals of nursing studies, and using research knowledge to promote an evidence-based practice.

You will need to read each chapter in your text before completing the chapters in this Study Guide. Scan the entire chapter to get an overall view of the content. Then read the textbook chapter with the intent of increasing your comprehension of each section. As you examine each section, pay careful attention to the terms that are defined. If the meaning of a term is not clear to you, look up its definition in the Glossary and identify other pages on which the term is used in the Index at the back of the textbook. Highlight key ideas in each section. Examine tables and figures as they are referenced in the text. Mark sections that you do not sufficiently understand. Jot down questions to ask your instructor in class or to post to your course discussion board.

After carefully reading a chapter in the text, complete the Study Guide exercises; this will assist you in learning relevant content. Each Study Guide chapter includes four major headings, which are discussed below.

Exercise 1: Terms and Definitions

This section of each Study Guide chapter consists of a matching test of key terms and their definitions. Key terms are listed at the beginning of each textbook chapter, and identified in color and defined within the chapter to assist you in becoming familiar with essential terminology for understanding the research process. By knowing these terms before you attend a class lecture on the content, you will be prepared to grasp the lecture content and perform well on course exams. As you read the text, do not skip over terms in the chapter that are unfamiliar to you. Instead, get in the habit of marking unfamiliar words as you read and looking up their definitions in the Glossary at the end of the text.

Exercise 2: Linking Ideas

This section of each Study Guide chapter helps you identify important information and link relevant ideas in each textbook chapter. Completing the fill-in-the-blank and matching questions will prompt you to review and analyze the content of the chapter, which is the key to comprehending and applying content related to the research process. You may need to refer to specific sections, tables, and figures in the text to complete some of these questions.

Exercise 3: Web-Based Information and Resources

Some chapters in the Study Guide include questions that require you to access online materials to answer the questions. These questions are provided to introduce you to the wealth of information that is available online related to research and evidence-based practice. Many of these resources are valuable websites that you may want to bookmark for use following graduation.

Exercise 4: Conducting Critical Appraisals to Build an Evidence-Based Practice

Critical appraisal exercises are provided to give you experiences in critically appraising published studies. In some cases, brief quotes are provided, with questions addressing information specific to the chapter content. The majority of the critical appraisal exercises focus on the three published studies that are provided in Appendices A, B, and C of this Study Guide. Two of the studies are quantitative and one of the studies is qualitative so that you can have experience in critically appraising both types of studies. The quantitative studies include one correlational type and one quasi-experimental type of study. On completing the Study Guide, you can incorporate the critical appraisal information you have learned to perform an overall critical appraisal of these three studies. In addition, you can take the knowledge you have gained and apply it in the critical appraisal of other published quantitative and qualitative studies.

Answer Key

The answers to all Study Guide questions are provided in the Answer Key in the back of the Study Guide. We recommend that you not refer to these answers except to check your own responses to the questions. You will learn more by reading the textbook and searching for the answers on your own.

Published Studies

Reprints of three published studies are provided in Appendices A, B, and C. These studies are referenced in many of the questions throughout the Study Guide. Additional published studies referenced in the Study Guide are found in the Research Article Library of the online resources for this textbook at https://evolve.elsevier.com/grove/understanding/.

Additional online questions and exercises (available at https://evolve.elsevier.com/grove/understanding/) have been developed to further enhance your understanding of the research process. You are now ready to begin your adventure of learning about the research process to build an evidence-based practice.

Contents

Angelico Marang

CHAPTER 1

Introduction to Nursing Research and Evidence-Based Practice

INTRODUCTION

You need to read Chapter 1 and then complete the following exercises. These exercises will assist you in learning key research terms, identifying the types of research conducted in nursing, determining your role in nursing research, and understanding evidence-based practice. The answers to these exercises are in the Answer Key at the back of the book.

EXERCISE 1: TERMS AND DEFINITIONS

Acquiring Knowledge and Research Methods

Directions: Match each term below with its correct definition. Each term is used only once and all terms are defined.

Terms

a. Borrowing
b. Deductive reasoning
c. Explanation
d. Inductive reasoning
e. Intuition
f. Knowledge
g. Nursing research
h. Outcomes research
i. Personal experience
j. Prediction
k. Qualitative research
l. Quality and Safety Education for Nurses (QSEN)
m. Quantitative research
n. Role modeling
o. Trial and error

Definitions

f 1. Information acquired in a variety of ways that is expected to be an accurate reflection of reality and is used to guide practice.

g 2. A scientific process that validates and refines existing knowledge and generates new knowledge that directly and indirectly influences nursing practice.

d 3. Reasoning from the specific to the general.

i 4. Gaining knowledge by being personally involved in a situation, such as providing care to patients in an intensive care unit (ICU).

m 5. A formal, objective, systematic research process to describe, test relationships, or examine cause-and-effect interactions among variables.

b 6. Reasoning from the general to the specific or from a general premise to a particular situation.

o 7. An approach with unknown outcomes that is used in a situation of uncertainty when other sources of knowledge are unavailable.

Angelica Martinez

e 8. Insight or understanding of a situation or event as a whole that usually cannot be logically explained.

k 9. A systematic, interactive, subjective research approach used to describe life experiences and give them meaning.

c 10. Knowledge generated from research that clarifies relationships among variables.

h 11. An important scientific methodology that was developed to examine the results of patient care.

j 12. Knowledge generated from research that enables one to estimate the probability of a specific outcome in a given situation.

l 13. An initiative that is focused on assisting students to develop the requisite knowledge, skills, and attitudes (KSAs) for each of the competencies for quality, safe pre-licensure education.

n 14. Learning by imitating the behaviors of an expert and the process of teaching less-experienced professionals by demonstrating model behaviors.

a 15. The appropriation and use of knowledge from other fields or disciplines to guide nursing practice.

Evidence-Based Practice Terms

Directions: Match each term below with its correct definition. Each term is used only once and all terms are defined.

Terms

a. Best research evidence
b. Clinical expertise
c. Critical appraisal of research
d. Evidence-based guidelines
e. Evidence-based practice

Definitions

e 1. The conscientious integration of best research evidence with clinical expertise and patient values and needs in the delivery of high-quality, cost-effective health care.

b 2. Knowledge and skills of the healthcare professional providing care; determined for a nurse by years of clinical experience, current knowledge of the research and clinical literature, and educational preparation.

a 3. The strongest empirical knowledge available generated from the synthesis of quality study findings to address a practice problem.

d 4. Rigorous explicit clinical guidelines developed based on the best research evidence available in that area.

c 5. Careful examination of all aspects of a study to judge its strengths, limitations, credibility, meaning, and significance.

Processes Used to Synthesize Research Evidence

Directions: Match each term below with its correct definition. Each term is used only once and all terms are defined.

Terms

a. Meta-analysis
b. Meta-synthesis
c. Mixed-methods systematic review
d. Systematic review

Definitions

d 1. Structured, comprehensive synthesis of quantitative and outcomes studies and meta-analyses in a particular healthcare area to determine the best research evidence available for expert clinicians to use to promote evidence-based practice.

a 2. Synthesis or pooling of the results from several previous studies using statistical analyses to determine the effect of an intervention or the strength of relationships that provides one of the strongest levels of evidence for practice.

c 3. Systematic synthesis of the findings from independent studies conducted with a variety of methods (quantitative, qualitative, and mixed-methods) to determine the current knowledge in an area.

b 4. Systematic compiling and integration of qualitative studies to expand understanding and develop a unique interpretation of the studies' findings in a selected area.

EXERCISE 2: LINKING IDEAS

How Research Influences Practice

Directions: The knowledge generated through research is essential to provide a scientific basis for the description, explanation, prediction, and control of nursing practice. Write a definition and provide an example of these four terms.

1. Description: ______________________________

____

____

Example: ______________________________

____

____

2. Explanation: ______________________________

____

____

Example: ____

____

____

3. Prediction: ____

____

____

Example: ____

____

____

4. Control: ____

____

____

Example: ____

____

____

Historical Events Influencing Nursing Research

Directions: Fill in the blanks with the appropriate word(s) or numbers.

1. ______________________________ is considered the first nurse researcher.
2. The first research journal published in nursing was ______________ ______________ and it is still considered one of the strongest research journals in nursing.
3. Many national and international research conferences have been sponsored by __________ __________ __________, the International Honor Society for Nursing to communicate study findings.
4. Identify three nursing research journals that were first published from 1978 to 1988.
   a. ____
   b. ____
   c. ____
5. The *Annual Review of Nursing Research* includes ____ ____.
6. The National Center for Nursing Research (NCNR) was established in ____________ by the National Institutes of Health.

7. The NCNR is now called the ______________________________.

8. The purpose of the National Institute for Nursing Research (NINR) is the ______________, ______________, and ______________ of information regarding basic and clinical nursing research.

9. ______________ was established in 1989 to facilitate the conduct of outcomes research and the communication of the findings to healthcare providers.

10. The Agency for Health Care Policy and Research (AHCPR) was renamed in 1999 and became the ______________________________. This agency is playing a major role in the development of evidence-based guidelines for use in practice.

11. The Department of Health and Human Services (DHHS) increased the visibility of and identified priorities for health-promotion research by publishing ______________________________.

12. The type of research that is focused on the quality and cost-effectiveness of health care that increased in the 1990s and continues to be strong today is ______________ ______________.

Acquiring Knowledge in Nursing

Directions: Fill in the blanks with the appropriate responses.

1. List five ways of acquiring knowledge in nursing, and provide an example of each.
   a. Traditions: Policy can have traditions, they can influence ~~the~~ in a positive way.
   b. Authority: When someone credits another as ~~source~~ source of Info.
   c. Borrowing: Integrating info from other disciplines within the focus of nursing
   d. Trial+Error: knowledge is gained from experience, it can fail.
   e. Role modeling: Admiring and imitating your favorite nurse.

2. Benner's 1984 book, *From Novice to Expert: Excellence and Power in Clinical Practice*, describes the importance of personal experience in acquiring nursing knowledge.

3. Identify Benner's five levels of experience in the development of clinical knowledge and expertise.
   a. Novice
   b. Advanced Beginner
   c. Competent
   d. Proficient
   e. expert

4. ~~Rea~~ Research knowledge provides an evidence base for the description, explanation, prediction, and control of nursing practice.

5. A "gut feeling" or "hunch" is an example of intuition, which nurses have found useful in identifying patients' serious problems.

Angelica Martinez

6. Traditions are based on knowledge of customs and past trends, such as providing hospitalized patients a bath every morning.

7. What type of reasoning is used in the following example? Deductive reasoning

   Human beings experience pain.
   Babies are human beings.
   Therefore, babies experience pain.

8. Identify three important outcomes that might be examined with outcomes research.

   a. Pt responses to nursing and medical interventions
   b. Pt satisfaction with the health outcomes, care recieved
   c. Maintainence of physical, mental, social functioning ~~of~~ for the pt

Linking Research Methods to Types of Research

Directions: Match the following research methods with the specific type of research.

Research Methods

a. Qualitative research method
b. Quantitative research method

Types of Research

b 1. Correlational research
b 2. Descriptive research
a 3. Ethnographic research
b 4. Experimental research
a 5. Exploratory-descriptive qualitative research
a 6. Grounded theory research
a 7. Historical research
a 8. Phenomenological research
b 9. Quasi-experimental research

Determining the Strength of Levels of Research Evidence

Directions: List the following examples of research evidence in order from the strongest or best research evidence to the weakest research evidence. The strongest research evidence should be a 1 and the weakest research evidence should be a 6.

_____ Single correlational study examining the relationships of body mass index, hours watching television per week, and hours on the computer each day.

_____ Systematic review used to develop the evidence-based guidelines for diagnosis and management of hypertension.

_____ Mixed-methods systematic review of qualitative and quantitative studies about effectiveness of medication administration technologies on medication errors.

_____ Meta-analysis of experimental studies (randomized clinical trials [RCT]) and quasi-experimental studies to examine interventions to reduce the weight of obese school-age children.

_____ Opinions of respected authorities on the management of diabetes.

_____ Single qualitative study of the process of weaning older adult patients from mechanical ventilation.

Nurses' Roles in Research

Directions: Match the levels of nurses' educational preparation with the research activities that each group of nurses is **primarily** responsible for according to the guidelines of the American Nurses Association (ANA) and American Association of Colleges of Nursing (AACN). It is acceptable to identify more than one nurses' educational preparation for some of the activities.

Nurses' Educational Preparation

a. Bachelor of Science in Nursing (BSN)
b. Master of Science in Nursing (MSN)
c. Doctorate of Nursing Practice (DNP)
d. Doctorate of Philosophy (PhD) in Nursing
e. Post-doctorate

Research Activities

_____ 1. Uses research evidence in practice with guidance

_____ 2. Develops and coordinates funded research programs

_____ 3. Critically appraises studies

_____ 4. Develops nursing knowledge through research and theory development

_____ 5. Participates in the development of evidence-based guidelines

_____ 6. Collaborates in conducting research projects

_____ 7. Conducts independent research projects

_____ 8. Critically appraises studies and synthesizes research evidence to develop and refine protocols and policies for a selected healthcare agency

_____ 9. Mentors PhD-prepared researchers

_____ 10. Coordinates research teams of BSN-, MSN-, and DNP-prepared nurses

EXERCISE 3: WEB-BASED INFORMATION AND RESOURCES

Directions: Answer the following questions with the appropriate website or relevant information.

1. Identify the current mission of the National Institute of Nursing Research (NINR). Search the NINR website for this information.

   ____

   ____

   ____

2. The Agency for Healthcare Research and Quality (AHRQ) has an excellent website that includes evidence-based practice guidelines at ______________________________.

3. Identify the website for the most current guideline for the management of hypertension (HTN):
   ______________________________.

4. Identify the website for *Healthy People 2020*: ______________________________

5. On the *Healthy People 2020* website, identify the website for Topics and Objectives on Adolescent Health:
   ____

6. Identify the website for Quality and Safety Education for Nurses (QSEN) competencies for pre-licensure nursing education: ______________________________

7. Search the QSEN pre-licensure nursing education website for the Evidence-Based Practice (EBP) Competency and identify this competency: ______________________________
   ____

   Also review the knowledge, skills, and attitudes (KSAs) listed for the EBP Competency.

EXERCISE 4: CONDUCTING CRITICAL APPRAISALS TO BUILD AN EVIDENCE-BASED PRACTICE

Directions: Locate the research articles (listed below) in Appendices A, B, and C. Review the titles, abstracts, and authors' credentials for these three articles. Identify the type of research conducted in each study.

Research Methods

a. Outcomes research method
b. Qualitative research method
c. Quantitative research method

Articles

_____ 1. Ågård, A. S., Egerod, I., Tønnesen, E., & Lomborg, K. (2012). Struggling for independence: A grounded theory study on convalescence of ICU survivors 12 months post ICU discharge. *Intensive and Critical Care Nursing, 28*(2), 105-113. (Provided in Appendix A)

_____ 2. Bindler, R. J., Bindler, R. C., & Daratha, K. B. (2013). Biological correlates and predictors of insulin resistance among early adolescents. *Journal of Pediatric Nursing, 28*(1), 20-27. (Provided in Appendix B)

_____ 3. Knapp, S. J., Sole, M. L., & Byers, J. F. (2013). The EPICS Family Bundle and its effects on stress and coping of families of critically ill trauma patients. *Applied Nursing Research, 26*(2), 51-57. (Provided in Appendix C)

Researchers' Credentials

Directions: Review the educational, research, and clinical credentials of the authors of the three research articles in Appendices A, B, and C. The articles include some information about the authors, but you can also search for the authors' credentials online.

1. Discuss whether Ågård et al. (2012) have the educational, research, and clinical preparation to conduct their study.

2. Discuss whether Bindler et al. (2013) have the educational, research, and clinical preparation to conduct their study.

3. Discuss whether Knapp et al. (2013) have the educational, research, and clinical preparation to conduct their study.

Study Titles and Abstracts

Directions: Critically appraise the title and abstract of the Bindler et al. (2013) study.

1. Critical appraisal of the title of the Bindler et al. (2013) study.

2. Critical appraisal of the abstract of the Bindler et al. (2013) study.

Directions: Post your ideas for the following on your Research Course Discussion Board. Look for input from other students and faculty.

1. Critically appraise the title and abstract for the Ågård et al. (2012) study.
2. Critically appraise the title and abstract for the Knapp et al. (2013) study.

Angelica Martinez

CHAPTER 2

Introduction to Quantitative Research

INTRODUCTION

You need to read Chapter 2 and then complete the following exercises. These exercises will assist you in learning the steps of the quantitative research process; identifying the different types of quantitative research (descriptive, correlational, quasi-experimental, and experimental); and reading research reports. The answers for the following exercises are in the Answer Key at the back of the book.

EXERCISE 1: TERMS AND DEFINITIONS

Directions: Match each term below with its correct definition. Each term is used only once and all terms are defined.

Terms

a. Applied or clinical research
b. Assumptions
c. Basic research
d. Control
e. Correlational research
f. Descriptive research
g. Design
h. Framework
i. Generalization
j. Interpretation of research outcomes
k. Limitations
l. Pilot study
m. Quantitative research process
n. Quasi-experimental research
o. Reading a research report
p. Research problem
q. Research purpose
r. Sampling
s. Setting
t. Variables

Definitions

m 1. Formal, objective, systematic process to describe, test relationships, and examine cause-and-effect interactions among variables.

s 2. Location for conducting research that can be natural, partially controlled, or highly controlled.

a 3. Scientific investigations conducted to generate knowledge that will directly influence clinical practice.

d 4. Imposing of rules by the researcher to decrease the possibility of error and increase the probability that the study's findings are an accurate reflection of reality.

r 5. Process of selecting a group of people, events, behaviors, or other elements that are representative of the population being studied.

c 6. Scientific investigations for the pursuit of "knowledge for knowledge's sake," or for the pleasure of learning.

Angelica Martinez

i 7. Extension of the implications of the findings from the sample that was studied to the larger population.

l 8. Smaller version of a proposed study conducted to develop and/or refine the methodology, such as the intervention, measurement instruments, or data collection process, to be used in a larger study.

q 9. The specific goal or focus of a study that directs the remaining steps of the research process.

K 10. Restrictions in a study methodology and/or framework that may decrease the credibility and generalizability of the findings.

n 11. Type of quantitative research that is conducted to examine causal relationships or to determine the effect of an independent variable on the dependent variable, but lacks the control of an experimental study.

o 12. Use of the skills of skimming, comprehending, and analyzing content from research reports.

f 13. Type of quantitative research that involves the exploration and description of phenomena in real-life situations.

t 14. Concepts at various levels of abstraction that are measured, manipulated, or controlled in a study.

h 15. The abstract, theoretical basis for a study that enables the researcher to link the findings to nursing's body of knowledge.

g 16. Blueprint for the conduct of a study that maximizes control over factors that could interfere with the study's desired outcome.

e 17. Type of quantitative research that involves the systematic investigation of relationships between or among variables.

j 18. Step in the research process that involves examining the results of data analysis, forming conclusions, considering implications for nursing, exploring the significance of the findings, generalizing the findings, and suggesting further studies.

p. 19. A step in the research process that identifies the gap in nursing knowledge needed for practice and indicates an area for further research.

b. 20. Statements that are taken for granted or are considered true even though they have not been scientifically tested.

EXERCISE 2: LINKING IDEAS

Control in Quantitative Research

Directions: Fill in the blanks with the appropriate word(s).

1. An experimental study is conducted in a(n) ______________________ setting.

2. Extraneous variables need to be controlled in ______________________ and ______________________ types of quantitative research to ensure that the findings are accurate reflections of reality.

3. ________________________________ and ________________________________ studies are usually conducted in natural settings and are not controlled to the same degree as other types of quantitative research.

4. ________________________________ studies need to include random assignment of subjects to the intervention and control groups.

5. Frequently, a(n) ____________________________ sampling method is used in descriptive and correlational studies. However, a(n) ____________________________ sampling method might also be used.

6. A subject's home is an example of a(n) ______________________ setting.

7. Laboratories, research units, and research centers are examples of ______________________________ settings where experimental research is conducted.

8. Researcher control is greatest in what type of quantitative research? ______________________

9. Hospital units are examples of ____________________________________ settings that allow the researcher to control some of the extraneous variables.

Steps of the Research Process

Directions: Fill in the blanks with the appropriate word(s).

1. The research process is similar to the ____________________________________ and the ____________________________ processes.

2. List the steps of the quantitative research process in their typical order of occurrence.

   Step 1 ____

   Step 2 ____

   Step 3 ____

   Step 4 ____

   Step 5 ____

   Step 6 ____

   Step 7 ____

   Step 8 ____

   Step 9 ____

   Step 10 ____

   Step 11 ____

Angelica Martinez

3. Assumptions are ____

____

____.

4. Identify three common assumptions on which various nursing studies have been based.

   a. ____

   b. ____

   c. ____

5. A pilot study is ____

____.

6. Identify two reasons for conducting a pilot study.

   a. ____

   b. ____

Reading Research Reports

Directions: Fill in the blanks with the appropriate responses.

1. The most common sources for nursing research reports are professional journals. Identify three nursing research journals.

   a. Applied Nursing Research

   b. Clinical Nursing Research

   c. World Views on Evidence-Based Nursing

2. Identify two clinical journals that include several research articles in each issue.

   a. Birth

   b. Heart and Lung

3. Identify the four major or primary sections of a research report.

   a. Introduction

   b. Methods

   c. Results

   d. Discussion

Angelica Martinez

4. The methods section of a research report describes how a study was conducted and usually includes:

 a. the study design
 b. treatment (if appropiate)
 c. Sample
 d. setting
 e. measurement methods

5. The discussion section ties the other sections of the research report together and gives them meaning. This section includes:

 a. the major findings
 b. limitations of the study
 c. conclusion drawn from the findings
 d. ~~tett~~ recommendations for further research
 e. Implications of the findings for nursing

6. The problem and purpose are often identified in which section of a research report? Introduction

7. The reference list at the end of a research report includes the relevant Studies and theoretical sources that provide a basis for the study and are cited in the report.

8. Reading a research report involves skimming, comprehending, and analyzing the content of the report.

9. In reading a research report, the comprehending step involves reading the study carefully. Focus on understanding major concepts and the flow of ideas.

10. In reading a research report, the analyzing step involves determining the value of the report's content. Break up the content and in depth, examine the parts for comprehension, accuracy and organization.

Angelica Martinez

Types of Quantitative Research

Directions: Match the type of quantitative research listed below with the examples of study titles.

Type of Quantitative Research

a. Descriptive research
b. Correlational research
c. Quasi-experimental research
d. Experimental research

Examples of Study Titles

c 1. Determining the effects of a relaxation technique versus standard care on patients' postoperative pain and anxiety levels.

a 2. Identifying the incidence of HIV in adolescents and young adults.

b 3. Examining the relationships among age, gender, knowledge of AIDS, and use of condoms by college students.

a 4. Describing the coping strategies of chronically ill men and women.

c 5. Determining the effects of position on sacral and heel pressures in hospitalized older adults.

d 6. Determining the effect of impaired physical mobility on skeletal muscle atrophy in laboratory rats.

a 7. Identifying current nursing practice behaviors for male and female nurses working in an intensive care area.

b 8. Examining the relationships among intensive care unit (ICU) stress, anxiety, and recovery rate for patients following cardiac surgery.

c 9. Examining the effects of a preadmission self-instruction program on patients' postoperative activity levels, anxiety levels, pain perception, lengths of hospital stay, and time until return to work.

d 10. Examining the effects of thermal applications on the abdominal temperatures of laboratory dogs.

b 11. Examining the relationships among hardiness, depression, and coping in institutionalized older adults.

a 12. Determining the incidence of drug abuse in registered nurses in community and hospital settings.

d 13. Examining the effect of warm and cold applications on the resolution of IV infiltrations in hospitalized patients.

a 14. Determining the stress levels and desired support of family caregivers of older adults with Alzheimer's disease.

c 15. Examining the effectiveness of breast cancer screening programs for women residing in rural areas.

a 16. Comparing the ages and coping skills of mothers pregnant with the first child in three ethnic groups (Caucasian, African American, and Hispanic).

b 17. Using age, nutritional intake, mobility level, weight, level of cognitive function, and serum albumin to predict the risk for pressure ulcers in hospitalized patients on a medical-surgical unit.

Angelica Martinez

a 18. Describing the severity of fatigue and anxiety in individuals with chronic obstructive pulmonary disease.

a 19. Describing and comparing the health-promotion and illness-prevention behaviors of African-American and Caucasian older adults.

b 20. Examining the relationships among the lipid values, blood pressure, weight, and stress levels of adolescents.

EXERCISE 3: WEB-BASED INFORMATION AND RESOURCES

Directions: Search for quantitative study information.

1. Search the Elsevier website for *Understanding Nursing Research*, 6th edition, http://evolve.elsevier.com/Grove/understanding, and find the following study: Farrell, G. A., & Shafiei, T. (2012). Workplace aggression, including bullying in nursing and midwifery: A descriptive survey (the SWAB study). *International Journal of Nursing Studies, 49*(11), 1423-1431.

   What type of study is this? ________________ Provide a rationale for your answer.

   ____

   ____

   ____

2. Search the Elsevier website for *Understanding Nursing Research*, 6th edition, http://evolve.elsevier.com/Grove/understanding, and find the following study: Aronson, B., Glynn, B., & Squires, T. (2013). Effectiveness of a role-modeling intervention on student nurse simulation competency. *Clinical Simulation in Nursing, 9*(4), e121-e126.

   What type of study is this? ________________ Provide a rationale for your answer.

   ____

   ____

   ____

3. Search the National Institute of Nursing Research (NINR) website and examine the types of research being conducted in nursing. Review the research in the "Research Highlights" section. What was the website you searched?

   ____

   ____

   ____

EXERCISE 4: CONDUCTING CRITICAL APPRAISALS TO BUILD AN EVIDENCE-BASED PRACTICE

Directions: Read the research articles in Appendices A, B, and C and answer the following questions.

Type of Quantitative or Qualitative Research

Directions: Identify the type of quantitative or qualitative research conducted in each study.

Type of Research

a. Descriptive research
b. Correlational research
c. Quasi-experimental research
d. Experimental research
e. Phenomenological research
f. Grounded theory research
g. Ethnographic research
h. Historical research

Study

_____ 1. Ågård, A. S., Egerod, I., Tønnesen, E., & Lomborg K. (2012). Struggling for independence: A grounded theory study on convalescence of ICU survivors 12 months post ICU discharge. *Intensive and Critical Care Nursing, 28*(2), 105-113. (Provided in Appendix A)

_____ 2. Bindler, R. J., Bindler, R. C., & Daratha, K. B. (2013). Biological correlates and predictors of insulin resistance among early adolescents. *Journal of Pediatric Nursing, 28*(1), 20-27 (Provided in Appendix B)

_____ 3. Knapp, S. J., Sole, M. L., & Byers, J. F. (2013). The EPICS Family Bundle and its effects on stress and coping of families of critically ill trauma patients. *Applied Nursing Research, 26*(2), 51-57. (Provided in Appendix C)

Type of Setting

Directions: Identify the type of setting for each study and provide rationales for your answers.

a. Natural setting
b. Partially controlled setting
c. Highly controlled setting

_____ 1. Ågård et al. (2012) study setting

Rationale: ____

____

____

____

_____ 2. Bindler et al. (2013) study setting

Rationale: ____

____

____

____

_____ 3. Knapp et al. (2013) study setting

Rationale: ____

____

____

____

Type of Research Conducted (Applied or Basic)

Directions: Indicate the type of nursing research conducted in each study.

Type of Nursing Research

a. Applied nursing research
b. Basic nursing research

Study

_____ 1. Ågård et al. (2012) study

_____ 2. Bindler et al. (2013) study

_____ 3. Knapp et al. (2013) study

Angelica Martinez

CHAPTER 3

Introduction to Qualitative Research

INTRODUCTION

Read Chapter 3 and then complete the following exercises. These exercises will assist you in learning key terms and reading and comprehending published qualitative studies. The answers for the following exercises are in the Answer Key at the back of the book.

EXERCISE 1: TERMS AND DEFINITIONS

Directions: Match each term below with its correct definition. Each term is used only once and all terms are defined.

Term

a. Bracketing
b. Ethnographic research
c. Ethnonursing research
d. Exploratory-descriptive qualitative research
e. Field notes
f. Focus group
g. Grounded theory research
h. Historical research
i. Participant
j. Phenomenology
k. Qualitative research
l. Rigor
m. Secondary source
n. Transcription
o. Unstructured interview

Definitions

__o__ 1. Questioning research participants orally without a fixed list of questions.

__n__ 2. Typing a verbatim narrative from a recorded interview or focus group.

__l__ 3. Characteristics of study methods that give the findings credibility and greater value.

__d__ 4. Research based on a pragmatic philosophy and focused on increasing understanding or finding a solution.

__i__ 5. A person from whom data are collected during a qualitative study.

__m__ 6. Account of an event by a person who learned about the event from another person.

__k__ 7. Systematic, subjective approach to describe life experiences and give them meaning.

__f__ 8. Gathering data from multiple participants simultaneously to encourage interaction and discussion.

__j__ 9. Focused on the lived experience.

__e__ 10. Using Dr. Leininger's methods to describe a cultural group.

Angelica Martinez

e 11. Notes from a research observation.

g 12. Qualitative method that describes social processes and proposes a framework of related concepts.

h 13. Research of events in the past in which nurses played a role.

a 14. Setting aside one's values and perspectives during the data collection and analysis process.

b 15. Study that explores the culture of a specific group of people or an organization.

Definitions in Your Own Words

Directions: Define the following terms in your own words without looking at your textbook. Then check your definitions with those in the glossary of your textbook. Using this strategy, you can identify elements of the term that are not yet clear in your mind. Reread that section of the chapter to clarify your understanding of the term.

1. Observation: ____________________

____

2. Coding: ____________________

____

3. Researcher-participant relationship: ____________________

____

EXERCISE 2: LINKING IDEAS

People and Their Contributions to Qualitative Research

Directions: Match the names of people below with the correct description. Each name is used only once and all people are described.

Description

a. Philosopher associated with the interpretive approach to phenomenology.
b. Developed the Sunshine Model of Transcultural Nursing Care.
c. Philosopher associated with the descriptive approach to phenomenology.
d. Person who developed the symbolic interaction theory.
e. Early studies on dying led to the grounded theory method.

Names

_____ 1. Leininger

_____ 2. Glaser and Strauss

_____ 3. Husserl

_____ 4. Heidegger

_____ 5. Mead

Qualitative Research Methodology

Directions: Fill in the blanks with the appropriate word(s).

1. The researcher listens to the recordings of interviews several times and reads and rereads the transcripts to become ______________________________ in the data.

2. An ethnographer lives in a different culture for a year, learns the language, and slowly stops communicating with family and friends in her home country. When asked when she plans to return, the ethnographer says she has not decided because she prefers the culture here more than she does the culture of her own country. There is a danger that the ethnographer has "gone ____________________."

3. The observer writes down comments and descriptions of body language during the focus group. The observer is preparing __________________ ______________.

4. During a study of men living with chronic illness, the researcher asks the participant at the end of the interview if he knows other men with chronic illness. When he replies that he does, the researcher gives him flyers about the study to share with the men. The flyer includes the researcher's contact information in case the recipient is willing to be interviewed. This is an example of ________________________ sampling.

5. The researcher is gathering data through focus groups of African-American adolescents. The researcher selects an African-American nurse to lead the focus group. The role that the focus group leader will fill is being the __________________.

Approaches to Qualitative Research

Directions: Match each qualitative approach with its characteristics. Label them P, G, E, H, and/or ED according to the key below for each area. All answers will be used once. Some answers will be used more than once.

Characteristics

P = Phenomenological
G = Grounded theory
E = Ethnographic
H = Historical
ED = Exploratory-descriptive qualitative

Qualitative Approach

_____ 1. May use key informants in the study of cultures.

_____ 2. Refers to a philosophy and a research method.

_____ 3. Uses primary and secondary sources to study the past.

_____ 4. Seeks to develop a framework of concepts or theory.

_____ 5. Emerged from the discipline of anthropology.

_____ 6. Undertaken from a pragmatic perspective and for a specific reason.

_____ 7. Studies the meaning of a lived experience.

_____ 8. Develops an inventory of sources.

EXERCISE 3: WEB-BASED INFORMATION AND RESOURCES

1. What are the differences between quantitative and qualitative research? Find websites that provide comparisons of quantitative and qualitative research. One such website is the page of the University of Wisconsin-Madison:

   URL: http://researchguides.ebling.library.wisc.edu/nursing

   Directions: Use the websites you find to complete the table with differences in quantitative and qualitative research.

Qualitative	Quantitative

Angelica Martinez

Directions: The online resource library includes three qualitative studies (Fry, 2011; Harvey, Kovalesky, Woods, & Loan, 2013; Wallace & Storm, 2007). Read the abstracts of the three articles and complete the following information.

Fry (2011)

Study Characteristic	Answer
Country/state in which the study was conducted.	Australia
Identify the qualitative approaches used (phenomenology, grounded theory, exploratory-descriptive qualitative, ethnography, historical).	Ethnography
Identify the human experience or topic of the study.	To understand how beliefs impact Austialian Emergency Department triage nursing practice.
Describe the sample.	10 Triage Nurse
How were the data collected?	200 hours of nonparticipant observation

Angelica Martinez

Harvey et al. (2013)

Study Characteristic	Answer
Country/state in which the study was conducted.	United States in Washington State
Identify the qualitative approaches used (phenomenology, grounded theory, exploratory-descriptive qualitative, ethnography, historical).	phenomenology
Identify the human experience or topic of the study.	Experiences of mothers of infants going through complex heart surgery.
Describe the sample.	8 mothers
How were the data collected?	• Joural entries with the mother's experience's. • Validation survey of 7 other ~~othe~~ mother's from a support group via email.

Wallace & Storm (2007)

Study Characteristic	Answer
Country in which the study was conducted.	
Identify the qualitative approaches used (phenomenology, grounded theory, exploratory-descriptive qualitative, ethnography, historical).	
Identify the human experience or topic of the study.	
Describe the sample.	
How were the data collected?	

EXERCISE 4: CONDUCTING CRITICAL APPRAISALS TO BUILD AN EVIDENCE-BASED PRACTICE

Directions: Read the Ågård, Egerod, Tønnesen, and Lomborg (2012) article in Appendix A of this study guide. Answer the following questions about that qualitative study.

1. What was the purpose of the study by Ågård et al.? ________________________________

2. Which qualitative method was used for the study? What rationale was given for using this method? __________

3. Look at Figure 1 and answer the following questions.

   a. How many potential patients and caregivers declined to participate? ____________________

   b. How many were excluded? ______________________________________

   c. Identify one exclusion criteria. ____________________________________

4. Describe the data collection process for the Ågård et al. (2012) study. ____________________

5. Table 1 in the article displays information about the patient participants. Use information in the table to answer the following questions.

   a. What was the shortest length of stay (LOS) in ICU for the patients? ______________________________

   b. Of the patients working prior to the ICU stay, how many were not working at the 12 month interview?

   ____

   c. Combining ICU, hospital, and rehabilitation stays, which patient had the longest stay in a health care facility?

   ____

6. The researchers expected to find that survivors would be experiencing psychological complications from their ICU experiences. What did they actually find?

____

____

7. Which quotation from a participant was most meaningful to you? Provide a rationale for your choice.

____

____

____

____

____

____

____

8. Ågård et al. (2012) identified several possible topics for future studies. Describe one below. ______________

____

____

____

____

____

____

____

____

CHAPTER 4

Examining Ethics in Nursing Research

INTRODUCTION

You need to read Chapter 4 and then complete the following exercises. These exercises will assist you in understanding the ethical aspects of a variety of nursing studies. The answers for these exercises are in the Answer Key at the back of the book.

EXERCISE 1: TERMS AND DEFINITIONS

Directions: Match each term below with its correct definition. Each term is used only once and all terms are defined.

Terms

a. Anonymity
b. Autonomous agent
c. Benefit-risk ratio
d. Confidentiality
e. Discomfort and harm risks
f. Ethical principles
g. Human rights
h. Individually identifiable health information
i. Informed consent
j. Institutional review
k. Nontherapeutic research
l. Plagiarism
m. Privacy Act
n. Research misconduct
o. Therapeutic research

Definitions

g 1. Claims and demands that have been justified in the eyes of an individual or the consensus of a group of individuals and are protected in research.

a 2. Condition in which a subject's identity cannot be linked, even by the researcher, with his or her individual responses.

i 3. Agreement by a prospective subject to participate voluntarily in a study after he or she has indicated understanding of the essential information about the study.

k 4. Research conducted to generate knowledge for a discipline; the results might benefit future patients, but will probably not benefit the research subjects.

j 5. Process of examining studies for ethical concerns by a committee of peers.

e 6. Phrase used to describe the degrees of risk subjects might experience while participating in research. These levels of risk include no anticipated effects, temporary discomfort, unusual levels of temporary discomfort, risk of permanent damage, or certainty of permanent damage.

m 7. Freedom of an individual to determine the time, extent, and general circumstances under which private information will be shared with or withheld from others.

Angelica Martinez

c 8. Ratio considered by researchers and reviewers of research as they weigh potential benefits and risks in a study to promote the conduct of ethical research.

o 9. Research that provides a patient with an opportunity to receive an experimental treatment that might have beneficial results.

f 10. Principles of respect for persons, beneficence, and justice, which are relevant to the conduct of research.

d 11. Management of private data in research in such a way that subjects' identities are not linked with their responses.

n 12. Practices such as fabrication, falsification, or forging of data; dishonest manipulation of the study design or methods; and plagiarism.

h 13. Any information, including demographic information, collected from an individual that is created or received by healthcare providers, health plan, or healthcare clearinghouse.

b 14. Humans who have the freedom to conduct their lives as they choose, without external controls.

l 15. The appropriation of another person's ideas, processes, results, or words without giving appropriate credit, including those obtained through confidential review of others' research proposals and manuscripts.

EXERCISE 2: LINKING IDEAS

Directions: Fill in the blanks with the appropriate responses.

1. List the elements of informed consent.

   a. Disclosure of essential study information to the study participant
   b. Comprehension of this info by the participant
   c. Competence of the participant to give consent
   d. Voluntary consent of the participant to take part in the study.

2. Identify the types of information that must be included in a study consent form.

   a. Intro of research activities
   b. Statement of the research purpose
   c. Selection of research subjects
   d. Explanation of procedures
   e. Description of risks and discomforts
   f. Description of benefits
   g. Disclosure of alternatives

Angelica Martinez

h. Voluntary participation

i. Option to withdraw

j. Consent to complete disclosure

3. Voluntary consent means that prospective adults with heart failure have decided to take part in the study of their own volition, without coercion or any undue influence, to improve their management of a chronic illness.

4. Subjects with diminished autonomy (e.g., the mentally ill or children) are vulnerable and incompetent to consent to participate in research.

5. A study conducted by a student must be reviewed by the Institutional review board of the University and the agency where data will be collected.

6. The three levels of institutional review of research are:

a. Exempt from review

b. Expedited review

c. Complete review

7. How do you assess the benefit-risk ratio of a published study? ______________________

8. What type of institutional review would a study probably require if it involved the review of patients' records to identify their fasting blood glucose values before surgery? ______________ ______________

9. A study that involved examining the effects of a new drug on patients' serum lipid values would probably require what type of institutional review? ______________ ______________

10. Identify three different types of research misconduct.

    a. ______________________________

    b. ______________________________

    c. ______________________________

11. The ______________ ______________ ______________ is a federal agency that was organized for reporting and investigating research misconduct.

12. Is research misconduct present in nursing? Provide a rationale for your answer. ______________

    ____

    ____

    ____

13. Are animals used in research conducted by nurses? Provide a rationale for your answer. ______________

    ____

    ____

    ____

14. What federal office was instituted to protect the welfare of animals used in research? ______________

    ______________ ______________ ______________.

15. What national organization was developed to ensure the humane treatment of animals in research? Many institutions have sought accreditation by this organization.

    ____

    ____

Historical Events, Ethical Codes, and Regulations

Directions: Match each unethical study listed below with the correct description.

Unethical Study

a. Jewish Chronic Disease Hospital Study
b. Nazi Medical Experiments
c. Tuskegee Syphilis Study
d. Willowbrook Study

Description

_____ 1. Subjects were exposed to freezing temperatures, high altitudes, poisons, untested drugs, and experimental surgeries.

_____ 2. The study was conducted to determine the natural course of syphilis in the adult black male.

_____ 3. Subjects were deliberately infected with the hepatitis virus in this study.

_____ 4. Subjects commonly were killed or sustained permanent physical, mental, or social damage during these studies.

_____ 5. Subjects did not receive penicillin when it was identified as an effective treatment for their disease.

_____ 6. The purpose of this study was to determine the patients' rejection responses to live cancer cells.

_____ 7. The subjects in this study were institutionalized mentally retarded children.

_____ 8. These experiments resulted in the development of the Nuremberg Code.

_____ 9. The patients and physicians providing care were unaware of the study, and it had not been approved by the IRB of the hospital.

_____ 10. This study continued until 1972, when an account of the study appeared in the *Washington Star* and public outrage demanded that the study be stopped.

Ethical Principles

Directions: Match the ethical principle with the example from research.

Ethical Principle

a. Principle of beneficence
b. Principle of justice
c. Principle of respect for persons

Example

_____ 1. A study focused on children age 7 to 16; they were given the right to assent to participate in the study.

_____ 2. The researcher developed a therapeutic study that would benefit the study subjects.

_____ 3. The subjects were given the right to withdraw from the study at any time.

_____ 4. The subjects were fairly treated by being randomly selected and assigned to a treatment or a comparison group.

_____ 5. The subjects were promised that an interview would take only an hour of their time, and the researcher kept to a schedule of hourly interviews.

Federal Regulations Influencing the Conduct of Research

Directions: Match the federal regulation with the content or definitions provided.

Federal Regulation

a. Department of Health and Human Services (DHHS) Protection of Human Subjects Regulations
b. Food and Drug Administration (FDA) Protection of Human Subjects Regulations
c. Health Insurance Portability and Accountability Act (HIPAA)

Content or Definition

_____ 1. Regulations provide direction for conducting research with pregnant women, human fetuses, neonates, children, and prisoners.

_____ 2. Regulations were developed to protect individually identifiable health information.

_____ 3. Regulations were developed in response to the Belmont Report.

_____ 4. Regulations are focused on clinical trials to generate new drugs and refine existing drug treatments.

_____ 5. Requires that an IRB or institutional privacy board act on requests for waivers or alterations of the authorization requirement for research.

Ethics of Published Studies

Directions: Match each ethical term with the appropriate example from a published study. You can read these studies on the Elsevier website for *Understanding Nursing Research*, 6th edition, at http://evolve.elsevier.com/grove/understanding.

Ethical Term

a. Coerced
b. Diminished autonomy
c. Fair treatment
d. Informed consent
e. Institutional Review Board review

Examples of Ethical Content from Published Studies

1. Aronson, Glynn, and Squires (2013) examined the effectiveness of a role-modeling intervention on student nurses' simulation competency. This study was approved by the university, which is an example of ________.

2. Aronson et al. (2013, p. e124) told the nursing students "that participation in the study was voluntary and that they would not be graded on their performance during the scenario." This is an example of ______ and ______.

3. Coker-Bolt, Jarrard, Woodard, and Merrill (2013, p. 64) conducted a quasi-experimental study that examined "the effects of oral motor stimulation on feeding behaviors of infants born with univentricle anatomy." The participants in this study were 28 infants (18 in the treatment group and 10 in the comparison group), who have ______ to participate in research because of their age.

4. Coker-Bolt et al. (2013) obtained permission from the families of the infants to involve them in their study. This is part of the ______ process.

5. Farrell and Shafiei (2012) conducted a study to describe workplace aggression, including bullying, for nurses and midwives. The nurses and midwives were given "the option to indicate if they agreed to be sent invitations to participate in the research." This statement indicates that the nurses and midwives were not ______ to participate in the study.

6. Farrell and Shafiei (2012) had individuals not involved in the study distribute the questionnaires to a random selection of nurses and midwives who consented to participate in the study. This indicates ______ of study participants.

EXERCISE 3: WEB-BASED INFORMATION AND RESOURCES

Directions: Fill in the blanks with the appropriate websites.

1. Identify the website for the Department of Health and Human Services (U.S. DHHS, 2009) federal regulations for the protection of human subjects in research.

   ____

   Review these regulations to determine how human subjects are protected during the conduct of research.

2. The ethical principles of respect for persons, beneficence, and justice were developed as part of the Belmont Report that guided the development of the DHHS regulations for the protection of human subjects in research. Locate the Belmont Report online:

   ____

   Review the focus of these three ethical principles.

3. Identify the website for the Food and Drug Administration (U.S. FDA, 2012) regulations for the protection of human subjects.

____

4. Locate the website of the HIPAA Privacy Rule that is focused on the information needed by researchers:

____

Review this information to determine how researchers protect study participants' private information.

5. Locate the website for the Office of Research Integrity (ORI), where the case summaries of research misconduct are discussed.

____

Review some of the case summaries and identify what types of research misconduct occurred.

6. Identify the website for the Office of Laboratory Animal Welfare (OLAW). _______________

____

Review the policies regarding the humane treatment of animals by researchers and institutions.

EXERCISE 4: CONDUCTING CRITCAL APPRAISALS TO BUILD AN EVIDENCE-BASED PRACTICE

Directions: Review the research articles in Appendices A, B, and C to answer the following questions.

1. Is the Ågård et al. (2012) study ethical? Identify the information in the study that indicates that the subjects' rights were protected through informed consent, HIPAA release, and institutional review of the study.

____

____

____

____

____

____

____

____

____

____

____

____

2. Is the Bindler et al. (2013) study ethical? Identify the information in the study that indicates that the subjects' rights were protected through informed consent, HIPAA release, and institutional review of the study.

3. Is the Knapp et al. (2013) study ethical? Identify the information in the study that indicates that the subjects' rights were protected through informed consent, HIPAA release, and institutional review of the study.

Angelica Martinez

CHAPTER

5 Research Problems, Purposes, and Hypotheses

INTRODUCTION

You need to read Chapter 5 and then complete the following exercises. These exercises will assist you in critically appraising problems, purposes, objectives, questions, hypotheses, and variables in published studies. The answers to these exercises are in the Answer Key at the back of the book.

EXERCISE 1: TERMS AND DEFINITIONS

Directions: Match each term below with its correct definition. Each term is used only once and all terms are defined.

Terms

a. Conceptual definition of variable
b. Demographic variable
c. Dependent variable
d. Extraneous variable
e. Hypothesis
f. Independent variable
g. Operational definition of variable
h. Research problem
i. Research purpose
j. Research question
k. Research topic

Definitions

d 1. Variables that exist in all studies and can affect the measurement of study variables; the researcher attempts to control the influence of these variables so they do not impact the study findings.

i 2. Clear, concise statement of the specific goal or focus of the study that is generated from the problem.

h 3. Area of concern or gap in the knowledge base that is needed for practice and thus requires study.

g 4. Description of how variables will be measured or manipulated in a study.

j 5. Concise interrogative statement developed to direct a study; focuses on description of variables, examination of relationships among variables, and determination of differences among two or more groups.

k 6. Concept or broad problem area that provides the basis for generating numerous research problems.

f 7. The intervention or treatment that is manipulated or varied by the researcher to create an effect on the dependent variable.

e 8. Formal statement of the expected relationship between or expected outcome from two or more variables in a specified population.

Angelica Marting

a 9. Definition that provides a variable or concept with connotative (abstract, comprehensive, theoretical) meaning; established through concept analysis, concept derivation, concept synthesis, or qualitative studies.

c 10. The response, behavior, or outcome that is predicted or explained in research; changes in this variable are presumed to be caused by the independent variable.

b 11. Variables that are identified and data that are collected from the study subjects so the sample can be described.

Types of Hypotheses

Directions: Match each type of hypothesis with the correct definition.

Type of Hypothesis

a. Associative hypothesis
b. Causal hypothesis
c. Complex hypothesis
d. Directional hypothesis
e. Nondirectional hypothesis
f. Null hypothesis
g. Research hypothesis
h. Simple hypothesis

Definitions

h 1. Hypothesis stating the relationship (associative or causal) between two variables.

g 2. Alternative hypothesis to the null hypothesis; states that a relationship exists among two or more variables.

b 3. Hypothesis stating a relationship between two variables in which one variable (independent variable) is thought to cause or determine the presence of the other variable (dependent variable).

e 4. Hypothesis stating that a relationship exists but not predicting the exact nature of the relationship.

c 5. Hypothesis predicting the relationships (associative or causal) among three or more variables.

a 6. Hypothesis stating a relationship in which variables that occur or exist together in the real world are identified; thus when one variable changes, the other variables change.

d 7. Hypothesis stating the specific nature of the interaction or relationship among two or more variables.

f 8. Hypothesis stating that no relationships exist among the variables being studied.

EXERCISE 2: LINKING IDEAS

Research Problem and Purpose

Directions: Fill in the blanks with the appropriate responses.

1. A clearly stated research purpose includes

    a. ______________________________,

    b. ______________________________, and usually the

    c. ______________________________.

Angelica Martinez

2. Research problems and purposes are significant if they have the potential to generate and refine relevant knowledge that:

   a. ______________________________

   b. ______________________________

   c. ______________________________

3. Identify two organizations or agencies that have developed lists of research priorities relevant to nursing.

   a. ______________________________

   b. ______________________________

4. The feasibility of a research problem and purpose is determined by examining the following:

   a. ______________________________

   b. ______________________________

   c. ______________________________

   d. ______________________________

5. Two ways to determine researcher expertise are by examining the ______________________ preparation and ______________________ experience of the researchers.

Understanding Hypotheses

Directions: Ten sample hypotheses are presented in this section. Identify each hypothesis using the terms listed below. Four terms are needed to identify each hypothesis. The correct answer for hypothesis #1 is provided as an example.

Terms

a. Associative hypothesis
b. Causal hypothesis
c. Complex hypothesis
d. Directional hypothesis
e. Nondirectional hypothesis
f. Null hypothesis
g. Research hypothesis
h. Simple hypothesis

Hypotheses

b, c, d, g 1. Relaxation therapy is more effective than standard care in decreasing pain perception and use of pain medications in adults with chronic arthritic pain.

a, c, e, g 2. Age, family support, and health status are related to the self-care abilities of nursing home residents.

b, c, e, f 3. Heparinized saline is no more effective than normal saline in maintaining the patency and comfort of a heparin lock.

a, d, g, h 4. Poor health status is related to decreasing self-care abilities in institutionalized older adults.

b, d, g, h 5. Low-back massage is more effective in decreasing perception of low-back pain than no massage in patients with chronic low-back pain.

_________ 6. Healthy adults involved in a diet and exercise program have lower low-density lipoprotein (LDL), higher high-density lipoprotein (HDL), and lower cardiovascular risk levels than adults not involved in the program.

_________ 7. Time on the operating table, diastolic blood pressure, age, and preoperative albumin levels are related to the increased development of pressure ulcers in hospitalized older adults.

_________ 8. There are no differences in complication rates or incidence of phlebitis between patients in whom heparin locks are changed every 72 hours and those in whom locks are left in place for up to 168 hours.

_________ 9. Nurses' perceived work stress, internal locus of control, and social support are related to their psychological symptoms.

_________ 10. Cancer patients with chronic pain who listen to music with positive suggestions of pain reduction have less pain than those who do not listen to music.

11. State hypothesis #2 as a directional hypothesis. ____

____

____

12. State hypothesis #5 as a null hypothesis. ____

____

____

Identifying Types of Study Variables

Directions: Match each type of variable with the sample variables provided below.

Type of Variable

a. Demographic variable
b. Dependent variable
c. Independent variable

Sample Variables

_____ 1. Age

_____ 2. Perception of pain

_____ 3. Exercise program

_____ 4. Gender

_____ 5. Length of hospital stay

_____ 6. Incidence of phlebitis

_____ 7. Anxiety level

_____ 8. Diet for calorie reduction

_____ 9. Educational level

_____ 10. Low-back massage

_____ 11. Relaxation therapy

_____ 12. Postoperative pain

_____ 13. Ethnic background

_____ 14. Total cholesterol value

_____ 15. Marital status

Understanding Study Variables

Directions: Match each of these terms concerning variables with the appropriate example.

Terms

a. Conceptual definition
b. Demographic variables
c. Dependent variables
d. Extraneous variable
e. Independent variable
f. Operational definition

Examples

_____ 1. Pain is a physiological and psychological response to a stimulus that occurs whenever and to the degree that a patient says it does. This is an example of what type of definition?

_____ 2. When you are examining the effects of nasal oxygen on oral temperature, you should eliminate all patients with fever from the study because fever has potential to affect the study's findings. This is an example of what type of variable?

_____ 3. The patients' pain will be measured using a visual analog scale and the Perception of Pain Likert Scale. This is an example of what type of definition?

_____ 4. The variables of heart rate, blood pressure, and respiratory rate are measured after the completion of an exercise program.

_____ 5. A patient receives a study intervention or treatment of ambulating every 2 hours.

_____ 6. Variables such as age, gender, ethnic origin, marital status, and medical diagnoses are measured to describe the sample.

EXERCISE 3: WEB-BASED INFORMATION AND RESOURCES

Directions: The following questions require identifying and searching selected websites. Review the key information provided on the websites.

1. The Bindler, Bindler, and Daratha (2013, p. 25) study "was supported by Agriculture and Food Initiative Grant 2007-55215-17909 from the USDA [U.S. Department of Agriculture] National Institute for Food and Agriculture." Identify the website for the USDA National Institute for Food and Agriculture:

    ____

    ____

    Review the types of grants offered by the National Institute for Food and Agriculture.

2. The references for the Bindler et al. (2013) study included the Centers for Disease Control and Prevention (2010). Identify the home page for the Centers for Disease Control (CDC):

    ____

    ____

    Review the type of information covered on this website.

3. On the CDC website, search for the topic "Childhood Overweight and Obesity." Identify the website for this topic.

____

4. Identify the website that provides "Strategies and Solutions" for the management of childhood overweight and obesity problems on the CDC website.

____

5. Locate the Coker-Bolt, Jarrard, Woodard, and Merrill (2013) study of "The Effects of Oral Motor Stimulation on Feeding Behaviors of Infants Born with Univentricle Anatomy" on the Elsevier website for *Understanding Nursing Research*, 6th edition, at http://evolve.elsevier.com/grove/understanding.

   a. Identify the research topics for this study. ____

   ____

   b. Identify the purpose of this study provided in the article abstract. ____

   ____

   c. Is the purpose complete or incomplete? Provide a rationale for your answer. ____

   ____

EXERCISE 4: CONDUCTING CRITICAL APPRAISALS TO BUILD AN EVIDENCE-BASED PRACTICE

Problem and Purpose

Bindler, Bindler, and Daratha (2013) Study

Directions: Review the Bindler et al. (2013) research article in Appendix B and answer the following questions.

1. State the problem of this study.

   a. Significance: ____

   ____

   ____

   ____

   ____

   b. Background: ____

   ____

   ____

   ____

   ____

c. Problem statement: ______________________________

2. State the purpose of this study. ______________________________

3. Are the problem and the purpose significant? Provide a rationale for your answer. ______________________________

4. Does the purpose identify the variables, population, and setting for this study? ______________________________

   a. Identify the variables. ______________________________

   b. Identify the population. ______________________________

   c. Identify the setting. ______________________________

5. Is it feasible for the researchers to study the problem and purpose? Provide a rationale. ______________________________

Knapp, Sole, and Byers (2013) Study

Directions: Review the Knapp et al. (2013) research article in Appendix C and answer the following questions.

1. State the problem of this study.

   a. Significance: ______

   b. Background: ______

   c. Problem statement: ______

2. State the purpose of this study.

   a. Purpose: ______

   b. Is this study purpose clear? Provide a rationale for your answer. ______

   c. Clearly state the study purpose. ______

3. Are the problem and the purpose significant? Provide a rationale.

4. Does the purpose identify the variables, population, and setting for this study?

   a. Identify the variables.

   b. Identify the population.

   c. Identify the setting.

5. Is it feasible for the researchers to study the problem and purpose? Provide a rationale.

Ågård, Egerod, Tønnesen, and Lomborg (2012) Study

Directions: Review the Ågård et al. (2012) research article in Appendix A and answer the following questions.

1. State the problem of this study.

   a. Significance:

b. Background:

c. Problem statement:

2. State the purpose of this study.

3. Are the problem and the purpose significant? Provide a rationale.

4. Does the purpose identify the concepts or variables, population, and setting for this study?

a. Identify the research concepts.

b. Identify the populations.

c. Identify the setting.

5. Is it feasible for the researcher to study the problem and purpose? Provide a rationale.

Objectives, Questions, and Hypotheses

Bindler et al. (2013) Research Article

Directions: Review this study in Appendix B and answer the following questions.

1. Are objectives, questions, or hypotheses stated in this study? Identify them.______________________________

2. Are they appropriate and clearly stated? Provide a rationale for your answer.______________________________

Knapp et al. (2013) Research Article

Directions: Review this study in Appendix C and answer the following questions.

1. Are objectives, questions, or hypotheses stated in this study? Identify them.______________________________

2. a. Are they appropriate and clearly stated? Provide a rationale for your answer. ______________________________

b. State a hypothesis for this study. ______________________________

____

____

Ågård et al. (2012) Study

Directions: Review this study in Appendix A and answer the following questions.

1. Are objectives, questions, or hypotheses stated in this study? Identify them.______________________________

____

2. Are they appropriate and clearly stated? ______________________________

Study Variables or Concepts*

Bindler et al. (2013) Study

Directions: Review this study in Appendix B and answer the following questions.

1. List the major variables in this study and identify the type of each variable (independent, dependent, or research).

Variable	Type of variable

*Ågård et al. (2012) study concepts are discussed in Chapter 3 of this study guide.

2. Identify the conceptual and operational definitions for the dependent variable *Homeostasis Model Assessment of Insulin Resistance* (HOMA-IR).

   a. Conceptual definition: ______________________________

   b. Operational definition: ______________________________

3. Are these definitions clear? Provide a rationale. ______________________________

4. Identify the demographic variables in the study. ______________________________

Knapp et al. (2013) Study

Directions: Review this study in Appendix C and answer the following questions.

1. List the variables in this article and identify the type of each variable (independent, dependent, or research).

Variable	Type of variable

2. Identify the conceptual and operational definitions for the dependent variable *stress*.

   a. Conceptual definition of stress: ______________________________

   b. Operational definition of stress: ______________________________

Identify the conceptual and operational definitions for the dependent variable *coping*.

c. Conceptual definition of coping: ______________________________

____

d. Operational definition of coping: ______________________________

____

3. Are these definitions clear? Provide a rationale for your answer. ______________________________

____

____

____

____

____

____

4. Identify the demographic variables in the study. ______________________________

____

____

____

____

Angelica Martinez

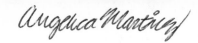

CHAPTER 6

Understanding and Critically Appraising the Literature Review

INTRODUCTION

After reading Chapter 6, complete the following exercises. These exercises will assist you in reading and critically appraising research reports and summarizing the findings for use in nursing practice. The answers for the following exercises are in the Answer Key at the back of the book.

EXERCISE 1: TERMS AND DEFINITIONS

Directions: Match each term below with its correct definition. Each term is used only once and all terms are defined.

Term

a. Article
b. Bibliographic database
c. Citation
d. Clinical journals
e. Conference proceedings
f. Data-based literature
g. Landmark studies
h. Peer reviewed
i. Primary source
j. Reference
k. Relevant studies
l. Replication studies
m. Secondary source
n. Theoretical literature
o. Thesis

Definitions

m 1. Source whose author summarizes or quotes content from a primary source.

d 2. Periodicals that include research reports and nonresearch articles about professional issues and practice problems.

l 3. Repetitions or reproductions of a study undertaken to determine if the results are the same in different settings or with different samples.

n 4. Literature that includes concept analyses, conceptual maps, theories, and conceptual frameworks that support a selected research problem and purpose.

h 5. Papers that were evaluated by other scholars as being of high quality, trustworthy, and acceptable for publication.

i 6. Source whose author originated or is responsible for generating the ideas published.

c 7. Paraphrasing or quoting content from a source, using it as an example, or presenting it as support for a position taken.

__a__ 8. A paper about a specific topic published together with similar documents on similar themes in journals, encyclopedias, or edited books.

__k__ 9. Research that has a direct bearing on the study being planned or topic of concern.

__J__ 10. The author, year, title of a source, and publication information that allows a reader to find the publication to which the author is referring.

__b__ 11. Compilations of citations and references that are searchable and allow the researcher to find articles and other publications on a specific topic.

__o__ 12. A research project completed by a student as part of the requirements for a master's degree.

__f__ 13. Reports of research studies that are published in journals, books, dissertations, and theses.

__e__ 14. Compilations of abstracts and papers presented at a professional meeting that may include the findings of pilot studies and preliminary studies.

__g__ 15. Significant research projects that influenced a discipline and led to the development of additional studies on the topic.

EXERCISE 2: LINKING IDEAS

Examples of Main Ideas from the Chapter

Directions: Fill in the blanks with the appropriate word(s)/response(s).

1. The process of reviewing the literature has three components, which are (1) finding __________________ research reports; (2) ________________________ ________________________ the studies; and (3) ____________________________ the study results.

2. The review of the literature identifies what is ____________________ and what is _______ __________ about a specific topic.

3. The bibliographic database most frequently used by nurses is ______________________________.

4. Current sources for a literature review are defined as those that were published within _____ years of when the article was accepted for publication.

5. The literature review is conducted at the beginning of the research process to direct the planning and implementing of a(n) ______________________ study.

6. The purpose and timing of the literature review for ____________________________ studies (qualitative approach) is very similar to the purpose and timing of the review for quantitative studies.

7. A well-written summary of a review of the literature provides direction for the formation of the ____________ of the study.

8. A(n) _________________________ is an alphabetized list of topics, each with a compilation of authoritative information on the topic.

9. Although information is readily available online, not all of the information websites provide is _____________ and __________________________.

10. The title of a journal article in a reference list that is formatted according to the American Psychological Association (APA) format will be in ______________________________ font while the name of the journal and its volume will be in ________________ font.

Theoretical and Empirical Sources

Directions: Theoretical and empirical sources are included in the literature review of a published study. Read the sources below and label each with a **T** if it is a theoretical source or an **E** if it is an empirical source. The final determination of the type of source would be made by reviewing the source.

_____ 1. Watson, J. (2008). *Nursing. The philosophy and science of caring* (revised ed.). Boulder, CO: University Press of Colorado.

_____ 2. Abstracts from the Southern Nursing Research Society Conference

_____ 3. Master's thesis

_____ 4. Jackson, J. R., Clements, P. T., Averill, J. B., & Zimbro, K. (2009). Patterns of knowing: Proposing a theory for nursing leadership. *Nursing Economic$, 27*(3), 149-159.

_____ 5. Orem, D. E., Taylor, S., & Renpenning, K. M. (2001). *Nursing: Concepts of practice* (6th ed.) St. Louis: Mosby.

_____ 6. Sammarco, A., & Konecny, L. M. (2010). Quality of life, social support, and uncertainty among Latina and Caucasian breast cancer survivors: A comparative study. *Oncology Nursing Forum, 37*(1), 93-99.

_____ 7. Raines, D. (2013). Mothers' stressor as day of discharge from the NICU approaches. *Advances in Neonatal Care, 13*(3), 181-187.

_____ 8. Doctoral dissertation

_____ 9. von Bertalanffy, L. (1968). *General systems theory*. New York: Braziller.

_____ 10. Rodwell, J., & Demir, D. (2012). Psychological consequences of bullying for hospital and aged care nurses. *International Nursing Review, 59*(4), 539-546.

Primary and Secondary Sources

Directions: A literature review includes mainly primary sources. Remember that a primary source is developed by the person conducting the research or developing the theory. A secondary source is the synthesis of primary and other sources. Based on these definitions, determine if a source is primary or secondary. Label each source below with a **P** if it is a primary source or an **S** if it is a secondary source.

_____ 1. Compilation of theories of management

_____ 2. Doctoral dissertation

_____ 3. Theory published by the theorist

_____ 4. Report of a pilot study to test the feasibility of an intervention

_____ 5. Seminal study comparing interventions for stress

_____ 6. Study published in *Applied Nursing Research*

_____ 7. Review of studies to develop an evidence-based practice recommendation

_____ 8. Published review of literature article

_____ 9. Exact replication of a study

_____ 10. Historical research article in *Image: Journal of Nursing Scholarship*

EXERCISE 3: WEB-BASED INFORMATION AND RESOURCES

1. Several websites are available as resources for individual nursing theorists. Search the International Orem Society's webpage (http://www.orem-society.com/) to fill in the answers to the following questions.

   In the journal *Self Care & Dependent Care Nursing: The Official Journal of the Orem International Society*, available through the Orem Society webpage, find volume 20 and the article by White. From the abstract, fill in the name of the midrange theory that White developed by extending Orem's theory with a new construct. Include the reference for the White article in APA format.

   Hint: Use the Publication tab and look on the left side of the page for the IOS Journal link.

   ____

   ____

   ____

   ____

   ____

   ____

2. Use Google Scholar (http://scholar.google.com/) to find the article by Smile, Dupuis, MacArthur, Roberts, and Fehlings published in 2013 about autism in children with cerebral palsy. From the abstract that is available for no charge, answer the following questions.

   a. Name the study design as identified by the researchers. ______________________________

   ____

   b. What was the median age of the children in the study? ______________________________

EXERCISE 4: CONDUCTING CRITICAL APPRAISALS TO BUILD AN EVIDENCE-BASED PRACTICE

Directions: Review the following three articles in Appendices A, B, and C: Ågård, Egerod, Tønnesen, and Lomborg (2012); Bindler, Bindler, and Daratha (2013); and Knapp, Sole, and Byers (2013). Use these articles to answer the following questions.

1. The most common way references are cited in nursing publications is APA format (*Publication Manual of the American Psychological Association*, 6th ed., 2010). Knowing the different parts of a reference citation will assist you in locating and recording sources for a formal paper. Please note that APA allows, but does not require, an issue number when a journal has continuous pagination across issues, meaning that the page numbers for Issue 3

begin where the page numbers for Issue 2 end. For example, in *Applied Nursing Research*, the last article in Issue 1 ended on page 48. The first article in Issue 2 started on page 49. In *Understanding Nursing Research*, 6th edition, and this study guide, we have chosen to include issue numbers whenever possible, because we have found that knowing the issue number can make finding an electronic article easier. You will notice the reference lists for the study examples may not include an issue number.

The following source is presented in APA format:

> Knapp, S. J., Sole, M. L., & Byers, J. F. (2013). The EPICS Family Bundle and its effects on stress and coping of families of critically ill trauma patients. *Applied Nursing Research, 26*(2), 51-57.

Please write the category of the citation information in the spaces provided.

a. In this reference, *Applied Nursing Research* is the ______________________________.

b. In this reference, 2013 is the ______________________________.

c. In this reference, 26 is the ______________________________.

d. In this reference, 51-57 refers to the ______________________________.

e. In this reference, 2 represents the ______________________________.

f. Who is the primary or lead author of this article? ______________________________

g. What is the title of the article? ______________________________

____

2. Write the reference for the Bindler, Bindler, and Daratha (2013) article using APA (2009) format. ____________

____

____

3. Incomplete and incorrect references in published studies are a problem for individuals trying to locate sources from the reference list of the article. The following reference citations from Bindler, Bindler, and Daratha (2013) article have had at least one element removed. Indicate what is missing and the part of the reference. For example, in the following reference, 2013 is missing, which is the year of publication.

> Knapp, S. J. , Sole, M. L., & Byers, J. F. The EPICS Family Bundle and its effects on stress and coping of families of critically ill trauma patients. *Applied Nursing Research, 26*(2), 51-57.

a. Moran, A., Jacobs, D., Steinberger, J., Hong, C. P., Prineas, R., Luepker, R., et al. (1999). Insulin resistance during puberty: Results from clamp studies in 357 children. *Diabetes, 48.*

What is missing?______________________________

____

b. Falkner, B., & Daniels, S. R. (2004). Summary of the fourth report on the diagnosis, evaluation, and treatment of high blood pressure in children and adolescents. *44,* 387-388.

What is missing?____

____

c. Langsted, A., Freiberg, J. J., & Nordestgaard, B. G. (2008). *Circulation, 118,* 2047-2056.

What is missing?____

____

4. What sections of the following articles included the studies' literature review?

a. Bindler, Bindler, and Daratha (2013): ____________________________

b. Knapp, Sole, and Byers (2013): ________________________________

5. In the article written by Ågård, Egerod, Tønnesen, and Lomborg (2012) about their qualitative study, in which two sections did they incorporate the review of the literature?

a. ____

b. ____

6. In the Ågård et al. (2012) article, what sources were cited as support for using classical grounded theory methodology?

____

____

Directions: For the next series of questions, critically appraise the review of the literature of the Ågård et al. (2012) article using the following questions from your *Understanding Nursing Research*, 6th edition, textbook.

7. Inclusion of relevant literature

a. Did the researchers describe previous studies and relevant theories? ____________________

____

b. What other types of literature were cited? ______________________________

____

8. Critically appraise the currency of sources for the Ågård et al. (2012) study. Include all cited sources, not just those included in the review.

a. To evaluate whether the references are current, identify the number and calculate the percentage of citations that were published in the last 10 years. ____________________________
Identify the number and calculate the percentage of citations that were published in the last 5 years.

____

b. Are landmark, seminal, and/or replication studies included? ______________________________

____

____

9. Breadth of the review

a. Based on the journal in which they published in 2007 and the title of the article, what discipline are Davidson et al.?

____

____

b. In what journal was the article by Cuthbertson et al. (2009) published? ______________________

____

c. Does it appear that the author searched databases outside of CINAHL for relevant studies? Provide a rationale for your answer.

____

____

____

____

10. Synthesis of strengths and weaknesses of available evidence

a. Are the studies critically appraised and synthesized? You can assess this by noting whether the authors commented on the strengths and weaknesses of the cited studies.

____

____

b. Is a clear, concise summary presented of the current empirical and theoretical knowledge in the area of the study, including identifying what is known and not known? If so, provide the summary that includes the statement of the research problem.

____

____

____

____

____

c. Is the literature review organized to provide a logical argument and demonstrate the progressive development of evidence from previous research? Provide a rationale for your answer.

d. Does the literature review summary provide direction for the formation of the research purpose? Provide a rationale for your answer.

11. Conduct a critical appraisal of the literature review in the Knapp et al. (2013) article. Write a summary paragraph about the strengths and weaknesses of this literature review.

CHAPTER 7

Understanding Theory and Research Frameworks

INTRODUCTION

You need to read Chapter 7 and then complete the following exercises. These exercises will assist you in learning key terms and identifying and critically appraising frameworks in published studies. The answers for the following exercises are in the Answer Key at the back of the book.

EXERCISE 1: TERMS AND DEFINITIONS

Directions: Match each term below with its correct definition. Each term is used only once and all terms are defined.

Terms

a. Abstract
b. Assumptions
c. Concept
d. Construct
e. Framework
f. Grand nursing theories
g. Middle-range theories
h. Philosophies
i. Proposition
j. Scientific theories

Definitions

_____ 1. An abstract, logical structure of concepts that guides the development of the study and links the study findings to nursing's body of knowledge.

_____ 2. Truths or principles of being, knowledge, or conduct.

_____ 3. Thinking oriented toward the development of a general idea, without association with a particular instance.

_____ 4. Less abstract, more specific theories than grand theories that focus on particular patients' health conditions, family situations, and nursing actions and are often tested in quantitative research.

_____ 5. Statements that are considered true without testing.

_____ 6. Abstract theories that are labeled as conceptual models by some scholars.

_____ 7. Theories of genetics or pathophysiology that are supported by extensive evidence and whose relational statements may be called *laws*.

_____ 8. A term that abstractly names an object or phenomenon.

_____ 9. A statement that describes the relationships among two or more concepts.

_____ 10. A broader category of ideas that may encompass several concepts.

EXERCISE 2: LINKING IDEAS

Key Theoretical Ideas

Directions: Fill in the blanks with the appropriate word(s)/response(s).

1. A(n) ______________________________ is more specific than a concept and is defined so that it is measurable in a study.
2. The ________________________ ________________________ of a theory are tested through research.
3. Statements at the lowest level of abstraction presented in a quantitative study are referred to as _______________ ______________________________________.
4. Concepts are sometimes called the ____________________ __________________ of theories.
5. How are the conceptual definition and operational definition of a variable different? ______________________

   ____

   ____

   ____

   ____

   ____
6. How are grand nursing theories and middle-range theories different? __________________________________

   ____

   ____

   ____
7. Situation-specific theories are called ______________________________ theories by some scholars.
8. Linkages between variables that are discussed but not fully developed or stated by a researcher are called the ____________________ ______________________________.
9. The elements of theory are concepts and __________________ ___________________.
10. Swanson (1991) published a middle-range theory of __________________________.

Levels of Abstraction

Directions: Place the following terms in order from the highest to the lowest level of abstraction.

Variable
Construct
Operational definition
Concept

_____________________________ *(highest)*

____

____

_____________________________ *(lowest)*

Elements of Theory

Directions: Study the diagram below and answer the following questions in the spaces provided.

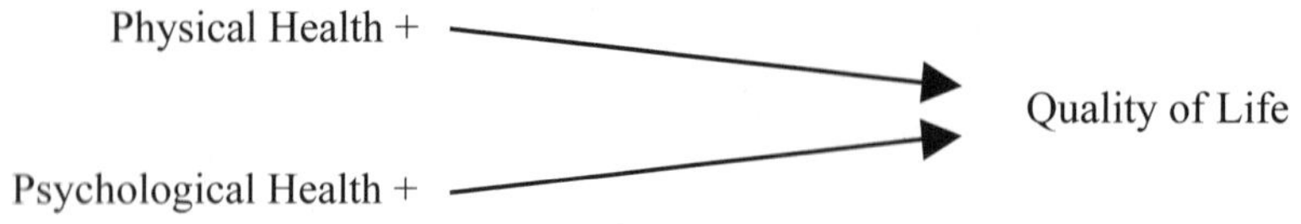

1. List the concepts in the diagram. ______________________________

2. What do the arrows represent? ______________________________

3. What does this figure represent when included in a study? ______________________________

Examples of Frameworks

Directions: Several theories were identified in Chapter 7 that have been used in studies. Match the name of the theory to the appropriate theorist's name. Hint: Review the middle-range theories in Table 7-4 in your textbook, *Understanding Nursing Research*, 6th edition.

Theorist(s)

a. Good and Moore
b. Jezewski
c. Kolcaba
d. Lenz, Pugh, Milligan, Gift, and Suppe
e. Mischel
f. Pender
g. Polk
h. Ruland and Moore

Theory

_____ 1. Acute pain

_____ 2. Comfort

_____ 3. Cultural brokering

_____ 4. Health promotion

_____ 5. Peaceful end of life

_____ 6. Resilience

_____ 7. Uncertainty in illness

_____ 8. Unpleasant symptoms

EXERCISE 3: WEB-BASED INFORMATION AND RESOURCES

Directions: Provide the appropriate responses for the following questions in the spaces provided.

1. Kolcaba developed the middle-range theory of comfort. Find a web page with information about her theory that includes the three types of comfort that she identified in 1991.

   a. Identify those three types of comfort: ______________________________, ______________________________, and ______________________________

   b. List the website where you found this information. ______________________________

2. Covell and Sidani (2013) published an article in volume 18 of the *Online Journal of Issues in Nursing* about Covell's Nursing Intellectual Capital (NIC) theory:

   Covell, C., & Sidani, S. (2013). Nursing intellectual capital theory: Implications for research and practice. *Online Journal of Issues in Nursing, 18*(2), Manuscript 2. **DOI**: 10.3912/OJIN.Vol18No02Man02. Retrieved from http://www.nursingworld.org/MainMenuCategories/ANAMarketplace/ANAPeriodicals/OJIN/TableofContents/Vol-18-2013/No2-May-2013/Nursing-Intellectual-Capital-Theory.html

   Developed from business and economic theories, the NIC theory includes definitions of different types of intellectual capital. Using the information in the article, match the concepts to examples of how the concepts can be operationalized or defined.

   ### *Concepts*

   Structural capital
   Intellectual capital
   Relational capital
   Human capital

   ### *Examples*

   a. Nurses' expertise and engagement loaned to the employer: ______________________________

   ____

   b. Knowledge translational strategies—how knowledge is shared: ______________________________

   ____

   c. Collective knowledge of an organization that shapes outcomes: ______________________________

   ____

   d. Practice guidelines and glucometers: ______________________________

   ____

EXERCISE 4: CONDUCTING CRITICAL APPRAISALS TO BUILD AN EVIDENCE-BASED PRACTICE

Directions: Read and conduct critical appraisals of the framework or theoretical sections of the following research reports.

Knapp, Sole, and Byers (2013)

Examine the concepts of the Knapp, Sole, and Byers (2013) study provided in Appendix C.

1. a. What nonnursing theory was the basis for the study? ____________________

   ____

   b. Who wrote the theory? ____________________

2. The intervention (the EPICS Family Bundle) was assumed to have an effect on which concept in Figure 1 in the Knapp article? *Hint*: The answer is near the end of the description of the theoretical framework.

   ____

Dickson, Howe, Deal, and McCarthy (2011)

Read the study by Dickson, Howe, Deal, and McCarthy (2011) available on the textbook website, http://evolve.elsevier.com/Grove/understanding/, and answer the following questions.

1. Five concepts were measured by the researchers (see Figure 1 of the Dickson article). The concept of decision-making was not measured. Fill in the table by providing the concept and variables for each construct. Some answers are provided to help you.

Construct	Concept	Variable(s)
Person		1. 2.
Problem	Job-level factors	1. 2. Job control 3.
Environmental	Work organization	Variables for this concept were not clearly separated from the variables for job-level factors
Behavior (implied construct)	Self-care	1.
Outcome (implied construct)		1. 2.

2. What theory did Dickson et al. (2011) cite for the conceptual definition for self-care on page 6 of the article?

   ____

3. What grand nursing theory could also have served as theoretical basis for this study? ______________________

____

Allen, Ploeg, and Kaasalainen (2012)

Read the Allen, Ploeg, and Kaasalainen (2012) article available on the textbook website, http://evolve.elsevier.com/Grove/understanding/, and answer the following questions.

1. For the two major concepts in the study, provide the conceptual definitions.

   Emotional intelligence: ____

   ____

   ____

   ____

   ____

   ____

   ____

   Clinical teaching effectiveness: ____

   ____

   ____

   ____

2. a. What mixed model did the researchers identify as the basis for one of their concepts? ______________

   ____

   b. Who developed the model? ____

3. Both of the concepts in the study had five sub-concepts as operationally defined. List the sub-concepts for each.

Emotional intelligence	Clinical teaching effectiveness
a.	a.
b.	b.
c.	c.
d.	d.
e.	e.

Bindler, Bindler, and Daratha (2013)

Read the article by Bindler, Bindler, and Daratha (2013) in Appendix B and answer the following questions.

1. What type of theory provided the foundation for the study?____

2. The researchers did not provide conceptual definitions for the variables. For each variable in the table below (not all the variables in the study), provide a conceptual definition and an operational definition in your own words. (*Note*: The operational definitions provided by the researchers are long, requiring several sentences. Summarize the operational definition as a short phrase using your own words.)

Variable	Conceptual definition	Operational definition
Obesity		
Serum lipids		

Piamjariyakul, Smith, Russell, Werkowitch, and Elyachar (2013)

Review the article by Piamjariyakul, Smith, Russell, Werkowitch, and Elyachar (2013) available on the textbook website, http://evolve.elsevier.com/Grove/understanding/, and answer the following questions.

1. In Figure 1 of the article, what did the solid arrows between coaching strategies and intermediate outcomes represent?

____

____

2. What is the meaning of the bottom horizontal box on the figure?________________________________

____

3. From the framework, two intermediate outcomes and one long-term outcome were measured. List the three variables measured related to the framework.

   a. ____

   b. ____

   c. ____

CHAPTER 8

Clarifying Quantitative Research Designs

INTRODUCTION

You need to read Chapter 8 and then complete the following exercises. These exercises will assist you in learning key terms and identifying and critically appraising designs in published studies. The answers for these exercises are in the Answer Key at the back of the book.

EXERISE 1: TERMS AND DEFINITIONS

Understanding Common Design Terms

Directions: Match each term below with its correct definition. Each term is used only once and all terms are defined.

Terms

a. Bias
b. Causality
c. Control
d. Correlational design
e. Cross-sectional design
f. Descriptive design
g. Experimental design
h. Longitudinal design
i. Multicausality
j. Nonexperimental design
k. Probability
l. Quasi-experimental design
m. Research design
n. Randomized controlled trial (RCT)

Definitions

_____ 1. Distortion of study findings that are slanted or deviated from the true or expected.

_____ 2. Blueprint for conducting a study.

_____ 3. Examines the effect of a particular intervention on selected outcomes.

_____ 4. Type of design that involves examining a group of subjects simultaneously in various stages of development, severity of illness, or levels of education to describe changes in a phenomenon across stages.

_____ 5. Study design that examines relationships between or among two or more variables in a single group.

_____ 6. The power to direct or manipulate factors to achieve a desired outcome. This is greater in experimental than quasi-experimental designs.

_____ 7. Descriptive and correlational designs are referred to as these types of designs since the focus is on examining variables as they naturally occur in the environment and not on the implementation of a treatment or intervention by researchers.

_____ 8. The recognition that several interrelating variables can be involved in causing a particular outcome.

_____ 9. Study designs to gain information about variables in relatively new areas of study, such as studies to identify problems with current practice or trends of illnesses, and categorize information.

_____ 10. Type of design focused on examining causality where extensive control of the intervention, setting, sampling process, and extraneous variables is possible.

_____ 11. Addresses relative rather than absolute causality.

_____ 12. Designs that involve collecting data from the same subjects at different points in time and might also be referred to as *repeated measures*.

_____ 13. Type of study currently conducted in medicine and nursing that is noted to be the strongest methodology for testing the effectiveness of a treatment or intervention due to the elements of design that limit the potential for bias. These studies usually are conducted in a single setting or in multiple geographical locations to increase the sample size and obtain a more representative sample.

_____ 14. Type of design that facilitates the search for knowledge and examination of causality in situations where control is limited in some ways.

Design Validity Terms

Directions: Match each term below with its correct definition. Each term is used only once and all terms are defined. Review the material in Table 8-1 in the textbook, *Understanding Nursing Research*, 6th edition, to expand your understanding of design validity.

Terms

a. Construct design validity
b. Design validity
c. Experimenter expectancy
d. External design validity
e. History
f. Internal design validity
g. Low statistical power
h Mono-operation bias
i. Statistical conclusion design validity
j. Threats to design validity

Definitions

_____ 1. Is a measure of the truth or accuracy of the findings obtained from a study and is focused on overall quality of the study design.

_____ 2. Threat to internal validity that occurs when an event not related to the planned study happens during the study that could have an impact on the findings.

_____ 3. Validity concerned with the fit between the conceptual and operational definitions of the study variables and the quality of the measurement methods used in the study.

_____ 4. Validity focused on determining if study findings are accurate or the result of extraneous variables.

_____ 5. Threat to construct validity where only one measurement method is used to measure a study variable.

_____ 6. Validity concerned with whether the conclusions about relationships or differences drawn from statistical analysis are an accurate reflection of the real world.

_____ 7. Threat to construct validity where researchers' predictions might bias or influence the outcomes of a study.

_____ 8. Problems that exist in a study design and need to be identified in critically appraising a study.

______ 9. Validity concerned with the extent to which study findings can be generalized beyond the sample used in the study.

______ 10. Threat to statistical conclusion validity that involves concluding there is no difference between samples when one exists.

EXERCISE 2: LINKING IDEAS

Directions: Fill in the blanks in this section with the appropriate word(s) or number(s).

1. According to causality theory, things have causes and causes lead to ____________________.

2. From the perspective of probability, a(n) ______________________________ may not produce a specific ____________________________ each time that particular ____________________ occurs.

3. Quasi-experimental study involves the manipulation of ______________________________.

4. Quasi-experimental and experimental studies are designed to examine ______________________________ ______________________________________.

5. The purpose of quasi-experimental and experimental research designs is to maximize ____________________________ of factors, such as extraneous variables, in the study situation.

6. The study design that has the highest level of control is a(n) ____________________________ ____.

7. Critical appraisal of research involves being able to think through threats to ____________________ ________________________ that have occurred and make judgments about how seriously they affect the integrity of the findings.

8. Hypertension is caused by a family history of cardiovascular disease (CVD), smoking, obesity, and lack of exercise, which is an example of ____________________________.

9. In studies examining causality, investigators implement a(n) ______________________________ that is expected to create a difference between the experimental and comparisons groups.

10. Developing a quality intervention and implementing it consistently in a study using a protocol promote ____________________________ ________________________ in the study.

11. A researcher wants to ____________________________ the design of a study by limiting the sample to only first-time elderly (>40 years) mothers.

12. Control is usually limited in ____________________________ and ____________________________ studies.

13. The ______________________ ____________________ design is used to examine descriptively the differences between two groups, such as the difference between males and females for surgical anxiety.

14. ________________________ studies are conducted to examine relationships among variables.

15. Middle-range theories, such as Selye's theory of stress and adaptation and Beck's theory of depression, are usually tested with ____________________ ______________________ designs.

16. List three elements of quasi-experimental and experimental designs that are focused on examining causality.

    a. ______________________________

    b. ______________________________

    c. ______________________________

17. Do randomized controlled trials (RCTs) usually have large samples ($N \geq 100$) or small samples ($N \leq 50$)? ______

Determining Types of Design Validity in Studies

Directions: Match the type of design validity with the examples provided from studies. The types of design validity might be used more than once.

Types of Design Validity

a. Construct design validity
b. External design validity
c. Internal design validity
d. Statistical conclusion design validity

Study Examples

_____ 1. A study had a large sample size and statistically significant relationships were found among body mass index (BMI), cholesterol values, and insulin resistance, which indicate what type of design validity?

_____ 2. Researchers and data collectors were blinded to the group receiving the intervention to strengthen this type of design validity.

_____ 3. Over 40% of the potential subjects approached declined to participate in a study because they did not want to participate in the intervention of a structured low-calorie diet. This interaction of the selection of subjects and the study intervention or treatment is an example of what type of threat to design validity?

_____ 4. The Beck Depression Inventory is a reliable measure of depression in research, which strengthens what type of design validity?

_____ 5. The subjects were allowed to select either the exercise (intervention) group or the no exercise (comparison) group in a study examining the effects of exercise on weight and cholesterol values, which is a threat to what type of design validity?

_____ 6. A study was conducted in three settings and all are supportive of research, which strengthens what type of design validity?

_____ 7. Only 10% of the subjects withdrew from a study because of the time constraints and personal and family illnesses, which strengthens which type of design validity?

_____ 8. A nutritional educational program was developed with precision and consistently implemented in a study, which strengthens what type of design validity?

_____ 9. The subjects were pretested and posttested in a study to determine a change in their nutrition knowledge following a nutritional educational program. However, the subjects noted they could remember the answers to several questions because of the pretest, which is a threat to what type of design validity?

_____ 10. Pain was measured with the Pain Perception Scale and FACES rating scale to strengthen which type of design validity?

Identifying a Design Model

Directions: Develop models of the appropriate designs in the spaces provided below. Refer to your textbook, *Understanding Nursing Research*, 6th edition, to help you with the different types of designs.

1. Typical descriptive design with four study variables:

2. Descriptive correlational design:

3. Quasi-experimental pretest and posttest design with comparison group:

Control and Designs for Nursing Studies

Directions: For each of the questions below, identiiy the **most** appropriate research design or study and provide a rationale for your answers. What elements might be controlled, if any? Each type of design or study is used only once.

Choices

Comparative descriptive design
Correlational study
Descriptive study
Model testing design
Predictive correlational design
Quasi-experimental posttest-only design with comparison group
Quasi-experimental pretest and posttest design with comparison group
Randomized controlled trial (RCT)

1. A study examined the effect on pain of showing a DVD of an animated program during the insertion of an IV in children 5-7 years of age. The study had experimental and comparison groups and a sample size of 80, with 40 children in each group. The subjects were obtained by a sample of convenience, with 40 children from one hospital unit and 40 from another unit. The children's pain scores were measured with the FACES pain scale immediately following the completion of the DVD and IV insertion.

___

___

___

___

2. A study was conducted to examine the effectiveness of a new drug to treat hypertension in adults. The study had a large sample of convenience and included all patients with hypertension in five primary-care clinics in two different cities in Texas. Subjects were randomly assigned to either the treatment group or comparison group. The drug intervention was highly controlled to ensure accurate delivery of the medication, and blood pressures (BPs) were precisely measured at the start of the study and 6 months later.

___

___

___

___

3. A sample of 100 first-time mothers was studied to examine the relationships among the variables of hours of sleep, stress level, anxiety level, and depression 1 month after the birth of their children.

___

___

___

___

4. The study included a sample of 80 patients experiencing their first myocardial infarction (MI). These patients were obtained by a sample of convenience from three cardiologists' offices. Subjects were asked to complete a questionnaire to identify their health promotion and illness prevention behaviors.

5. A study was conducted to describe and examine differences in health promotion behaviors for males and females with type 2 diabetes. The sample included 100 subjects—50 females and 50 males—who were obtained by a sample of convenience from two primary care clinics.

6. A study was conducted to examine the effect of vitamins on weight gain in a sample of infants who had failure to thrive at birth. The sample of 60 infants was obtained from three pediatricians' offices; 30 infants were randomly assigned to the experimental group and 30 to the comparison group. The infants were weighed before and after the implementation of the vitamin intervention, which lasted for 6 months. The intervention was implemented using a structured protocol.

7. The study was conducted to test the Orem Self-Care Model to predict the self-care behaviors of 50 diabetic adolescents. These adolescents were obtained from two school districts using a sample of convenience.

8. The study included a convenience sample of 80 women with lung cancer who were identified in three oncology centers. The women's perceived self-esteem, depression level, age, and educational level were used to predict their self-care levels. These variables were measured 3 months into the women's cancer treatments.

____

____

____

____

EXERCISE 3: WEB-BASED INFORMATION AND RESOURCES

Directions: Answer the following questions with the appropriate website or relevant information.

1. Search the Elsevier website for *Understanding Nursing Research*, 6th edition, http://evolve.elsevier.com/grove/understanding/, and find the following study: Farrell, G. A., & Shafiei, T. (2012). Workplace aggression, including bullying in nursing and midwifery: A descriptive survey (the SWAB study). *International Journal of Nursing Studies, 49*(11), 1423-1431.

    a. What type of design was used in this study? ______________________

    b. How were data collected in this study? ______________________

    ____

    ____

    ____

2. Search the Elsevier website for *Understanding Nursing Research*, 6th edition, http://evolve.elsevier.com/grove/understanding/, and find the following study: Aronson, B., Glynn, B., & Squires, T. (2013). Effectiveness of a role-modeling intervention on student nurse simulation competency. *Clinical Simulation in Nursing, 9*(4), e121-e126.

    a. What type of design was used in this study? ______________________

    b. Was an intervention included in this study? If so, identify the intervention. ______________

    ____

    ____

    ____

    c. Was the data collection process structured? Provide a rationale for your answer. ______________

    ____

    ____

    ____

EXERCISE 4: CONDUCTING CRITICAL APPRAISALS TO BUILD AN EVIDENCE-BASED PRACTICE

Bindler, Bindler, and Daratha (2013)

Directions: Examine the design of the Bindler, Bindler, and Daratha (2013) study in Appendix B, and answer the following critical appraisal questions about the design.

1. Identify the type of design used in this study. Provide a rationale for your answer. ______________________

____

____

____

2. What variable was predicted in this study? ______________________________________

   Is this variable an (**independent** or **dependent**) variable? *(Circle the correct answer.)*

3. In predictive correlational designs, independent variables are used to predict a dependent variable. What independent variables were used to predict the dependent variable IR in the Bindler et al. (2013) study?

____

____

____

____

4. What comparisons were made in the Bindler et al. (2013) study? ________________________

____

____

5. Identify three strengths of design validity in the Bindler et al. (2013) study.

   a. ____

   ____

   ____

   b. ____

   ____

   ____

   c. ____

   ____

   ____

6. Identify two threats to design validity in this study.

    a. ______________________________

    ____

    ____

    b. ______________________________

    ____

    ____

7. List two methods of control used in the Bindler et al. (2013) design.

    a. ______________________________

    ____

    b. ______________________________

    ____

8. To what population(s) can the findings from the Bindler et al. (2013) study be generalized? Provide a rationale for your answer.

    ____

    ____

    ____

Knapp, Sole, and Byers (2013)

Directions: Examine the design of the Knapp, Sole, and Byers (2013) study found in Appendix C, and answer the following critical appraisal questions about the design.

1. Identify the type of design used in this study. ______________________________

    ____

2. What intervention was implemented in this study? ______________________________

    ____

3. What comparisons were made in the Knapp et al. (2013) study? ______________________________

    ____

    ____

    ____

    ____

4. Identify two design validity strengths in the Knapp et al. (2013) study.

   a. ____

   ____

   ____

   b. ____

   ____

   ____

5. Identify three threats to design validity in the Knapp et al. (2013) study.

   a. ____

   ____

   ____

   b. ____

   ____

   ____

   c. ____

   ____

   ____

6. List three methods of control used in the Knapp et al. (2013) study design.

   a. ____

   ____

   b. ____

   ____

   c. ____

   ____

7. To what population(s) can the findings be generalized? Provide a rationale. ______________________________

____

____

____

____

____

____

Angelica Martinez

CHAPTER 9

Examining Populations and Samples in Research

INTRODUCTION

You need to read Chapter 9 and then complete the following exercises. These exercises will assist you in understanding and critically appraising the sampling process in published studies. The answers to these exercises are in the Answer Key at the back of the book.

EXERCISE 1: TERMS AND DEFINITIONS

Directions: Match each term below with its correct definition. Each term is used only once and all terms are defined.

Terms

a. Accessible population
b. Cluster sampling
c. Convenience sampling
d. Network sampling
e. Nonprobability sampling
f. Probability sampling
g. Purposeful or purposive sampling
h. Quota sampling
i. Simple random sampling
j. Sampling
k. Sampling criteria
l. Stratified random sampling
m. Systematic sampling
n. Target population
o. Theoretical sampling

Definitions

__j__ 1. Process of selecting a group of people, events, behaviors, or other elements that are representative of the population being studied.

__a__ 2. Portion of the target population to which the researcher has reasonable access.

__n__ 3. All elements (individuals, objects, events, or substances) that meet the sampling criteria for inclusion in a study.

__g__ 4. Judgmental sampling that involves the conscious selection by the researcher of certain subjects or elements to include in a study.

__k__ 5. List of the characteristics essential for membership in the target population.

__f__ 6. Random sampling occurs when every member (element) of the population has a probability higher than zero of being selected for the sample; example random sampling methods include simple random sampling, stratified random sampling, cluster sampling, and systematic sampling.

__m__ 7. Sampling method that involves selecting every *k*th individual from an ordered list of all members of a population, using a randomly selected starting point.

Angelica Martinez

i 8. Sampling method that involves random selection of subjects from the sampling frame for a study.

l 9. Random sampling method used when the researcher knows some of the variables in the population that are critical to achieving representativeness; the sample is divided into strata or groups using these identified variables.

b 10. Random sampling method in which a frame is developed that includes a list of all states, cities, institutions, or organizations that could be used in a study; a randomized sample is drawn from this list.

d 11. Snowballing technique that takes advantage of social networks and the fact that friends tend to hold characteristics in common; subjects meeting sample criteria are asked to assist in locating others with similar characteristics.

e 12. Nonrandom sampling in which not every element of the population has an opportunity for selection, such as convenience sampling, quota sampling, purposive sampling, network sampling, and theoretical sampling.

n 13. Convenience sampling method with an added strategy to ensure the inclusion of subjects who are likely to be underrepresented in the convenience sample, such as women and minority groups.

c 14. Sampling method that involves including subjects in a study because they happened to be in the right place at the right time.

o 15. A sampling method often used in grounded theory research to develop a selected theory through the research process.

EXERCISE 2: LINKING IDEAS

Directions: Fill in the blanks with the appropriate word(s)/response(s).

1. The individual units of a population are called ________________________.

2. The sample is obtained from the accessible population and is generalized to the ________________ ________________.

3. Representativeness means that the ________________, ________________ ________________, and ________________ ________________ are alike in as many ways as possible.

4. Identify two ways you might evaluate the representativeness of a sample in a published study.

   a. ________________________________

   b. ________________________________

5. Random variation is ________________________________ ________________________________.

6. A list of every member of a population is referred to as a(n) ________________ ________________.

7. A sampling plan outlines the ________________________________.

8. In critically appraising the sampling plan in a quantitative study, what three things might you examine?

   a. ______________________________

   b. ______________________________

   c. ______________________________

9. When the sampling criteria are narrowly defined or very specific, the sample desired is more ________________ ________________.

10. When the sampling criteria are broadly defined to include a variety of subjects, the sample desired is more ________________.

11. Subjects must be over the age of 18, able to read and write English, newly diagnosed with cancer, and have no other major illnesses. These are examples of ________________ ________________.

12. The sample was 65% female and 40% African American, 30% Hispanic, and 30% Caucasian, which are examples of ________________ ________________.

13. When 9 subjects were lost to a study due to complications ($n = 4$), hospitalizations ($n = 3$), and diagnosis of additional illnesses ($n = 2$), this is an example of ________________ ________________.

14. Identify four types of probability or random sampling discussed in the textbook, *Understanding Nursing Research*, 6th edition.

    a. ______________________________

    b. ______________________________

    c. ______________________________

    d. ______________________________

15. Identify three types of nonprobability or nonrandom sampling commonly used in qualitative research.

    a. ______________________________

    b. ______________________________

    c. ______________________________

16. Have the majority of published nursing studies to date used probability (random) or nonprobability (nonrandom) sampling methods? ________________

17. The adequacy of the sample size in quantitative studies can be evaluated using ________________ ________________.

18. Power is the capacity to detect ________________ or ________________ that actually exist in the population.

19. The minimal acceptable level of power for a study is ____________.

20. Effect size is a specific numerical value used to represent the extent to which the ________________ ________________ is false.

21. Identify three factors that influence the adequacy of a study's sample size in quantitative studies.

    a. ______________________________

    b. ______________________________

    c. ______________________________

22. Identify three factors that influence the adequacy of a study's sample size in qualitative studies.

    a. ______________________________

    b. ______________________________

    c. ______________________________

23. The two types of sampling criteria that might be included in a study are ______________________ and ______________________ criteria.

24. Calculate the refusal rate for a study in which 250 potential subjects were approached and 208 accepted participation in the study. What percentage of the potential subjects refused to participate?

    ____

25. Calculate the attrition rate for a study with a sample size of 150 and 20 subjects or participants withdrew from the study (10 due to increased morbidity, 5 due to time constraints, 3 due to transportation problems, and 2 due to mortality). What was the attrition rate for this study?

    ____

Sampling Methods for Quantitative and Qualitative Studies

Directions: Match the appropriate sampling method with the example sampling information from a study. Some answer choices are used more than once.

Sampling Method

a. Cluster sampling
b. Convenience sampling
c. Network sampling
d. Purposive sampling
e. Quota sampling
f. Simple random sampling
g. Stratified random sampling
h. Systematic sampling
i. Theoretical sampling

Examples

_____ 1. A sample of 500 nurses was randomly selected from a list of all registered nurses in the state of Texas.

_____ 2. A sample of 50 diabetic patients was obtained from an outpatient clinic and randomly placed in the comparison and experimental groups.

_____ 3. A sample of 10 subjects with HIV was obtained by asking three subjects to identify friends with HIV who might participate in the study.

_____ 4. A sample of 1000 critical care nurses was obtained by asking 100 critical care nurse managers in 50 randomly selected, large hospitals to identify 10 staff nurses to complete a survey.

_____ 5. A sample of 90 subjects was asked to participate in a study at an immunization booth in the mall.

_____ 6. Gender was used to stratify a sample of 100 randomly selected subjects.

_____ 7. The researcher obtained a list of all certified nurse practitioners, picked a random starting point, and then selected every 25th individual to participate in the study.

_____ 8. A sample of 120 hypertensive subjects was recruited in a clinic to participate in a study.

_____ 9. An equal number of patients with asthma, emphysema, and chronic bronchitis were recruited from the local Better Breathers Chapter and asked to participate in a study.

_____ 10. The sample included 24 patients; 12 were examples of strong self-care and 12 were examples of poor self-care.

_____ 11. A sample of 3000 military personnel was randomly selected to participate in a study.

_____ 12. A sample of 18 drug-addicted nurses was obtained by asking 7 subjects to identify friends who were drug-addicted.

_____ 13. A sample of 17 home health patients was asked to participate in a study because they had what were determined to be stage IV pressure ulcers that were not healing.

_____ 14. A sample of 150 adolescents was obtained at 3 fast-food restaurants.

_____ 15. A sample of 110 surgery patients was randomly selected from a hospital and randomly placed in control and treatment groups.

_____ 16. Starting from a random point, every 10th subject who entered the emergency department was selected for participation in the study until a sample of 100 was achieved.

_____ 17. A grounded theory study was conducted to develop a theory about responses to hurricane disaster, and a sample was selected to promote generation of the theory.

_____ 18. A sample of 120 heart transplant patients was obtained by asking 15 critical care nurse managers in 15 randomly selected, large urban hospitals to identify 8 patients to participate in a study.

_____ 19. A sample of 12 subjects who had experienced sexual assault was selected; 6 of them were considered to be coping well after the assault, and 6 were considered to be coping very poorly after the assault. Data saturation was achieved with these 12 subjects.

_____ 20. A sample of 150 subjects receiving care in a university health center was asked to participate in a study.

Determining Sample Size for Quantitative and Qualitative Studies

Directions: Match the type of research, quantitative or qualitative, with the criteria for determining the appropriate sample size for a study.

Type of Research

a. Qualitative research
b. Quantitative research
c. Both qualitative and quantitative research

Criteria

_____ 1. Sample size is adequate when saturation of information is achieved in the study area.

_____ 2. The scope of the study influences the sample size; a broad scope requires more subjects than does a study with a narrow scope.

_____ 3. Power analysis can be used to determine the sample size for the study.

_____ 4. The quality and the depth of information obtained from the study participants are used to determine the sample size.

_____ 5. As control in the study increases, the necessary sample size decreases.

_____ 6. The more sensitive the measurement methods used in a study, the fewer the subjects who are needed.

_____ 7. The more variables or concepts examined in a study, the larger the sample size that is needed.

_____ 8. The sample size needs to be large enough to prevent a Type II error.

_____ 9. Purposive sampling is a common method used to obtain an adequate sample size.

_____ 10. Simple random sampling is the strongest method of decreasing the potential for bias.

EXERCISE 3: WEB-BASED INFORMATION AND RESOURCES

Directions: Provide answers to the questions in this section.

1. Locate the Aronson, Glynn and Squires (2013) study titled "Effectiveness of a Role-Modeling Intervention on Student Nurse Simulation Competency" in the Article Library on the Elsevier website for the textbook, *Understanding Nursing Research*, 6th edition, at http://evolve.elsevier.com/grove/understanding/.

    a. What sampling method was used in this study? ____________________

    b. What was the sample size of this study? ____________________

2. Locate the Coker-Bolt, Jarrard, Woodard, and Merrill (2013) study titled "The Effects of Oral Motor Stimulation on Feeding Behaviors of Infants Born with Univentricle Anatomy" in the Article Library on the Elsevier website for *Understanding Nursing Research*, 6th edition, at http://evolve.elsevier.com/grove/understanding.

    a. What sampling method was used in this study? ____________________

    b. What was the sample size of this study? ____________________

    c. How many infants were in the treatment group? ____________ How many infants were in the comparison group? ____________

Angelica Martinez

d. Were the treatment and comparison group sizes a strength or weakness? Provide a rationale for your answer.

3. Search the Internet for "power analysis." Identify a website that discusses power analysis. Review the website to improve your understanding of power and power analysis in research.

EXERCISE 4: CONDUCTING CRITICAL APPRAISALS TO BUILD AN EVIDENCE-BASED PRACTICE

Bindler, Bindler, and Daratha (2013) Study

Directions: Review the Bindler et al. (2013) study in Appendix B to answer the following questions.

1. Identify the study population. Adolescents in middle school.
2. List the sample inclusion and exclusion criteria for this study. Inclusions students who volunteered to participate in a project called TEAMS. Exclusion criteria: students with mental or physical conditions or students taking insulin or taking oral glycemic medications
3. Identify the sample characteristics for this study. Increased IR, high-sensitivity C-reactive protein, triglycerides, and BP. Waist circumference and triglycerides were predicitive of IR.
4. What is the sample size? 150 Adolesants, 64 males and 86 females
5. Was the sample size adequate? Provide a rationale. The study should've been bigger to perform a power analysis to determine an good size for this study and groups studied

Angelica Martinez

6. What was the sample attrition for this study? Was this a study weakness or strength? ~~At~~ there was no sample attrition for this study. This would be a strength.

7. Was probability or nonprobability sampling used in this study? Nonprobability ~~m~~ sampling

8. What specific type of sampling method was used in this study? Convenience sampling

9. Was the sample in this study representative of the target population studied? Provide a rationale. No. There was way more girls than boys in this study, we would want an equal amount of boys and girls. The participants were also from a nonrandom sampling and only participants who volunteered to be in TEAMS.

10. Can the findings be generalized to the target population? Provide a rationale. Yes because this study is consistent with other studies. But more research needs to be done on this new ~~&~~ study to confirm that we can generalize this to the target population

11. What were the settings for this study? At their respective schools or at the university campus

Were the settings natural, partially controlled, or highly controlled? Natural controlled

Knapp, Sole, and Byers (2013) Study

Directions: Review the Knapp et al. (2013) study in Appendix C to answer the following questions.

1. Identify the study population. ____________________

2. List the sample criteria for this study. ____________________

3. Identify the sample characteristics for this study. ____________________

4. What was the sample size? ____________________

5. Was a power analysis conducted to determine sample size needed for the study? If so, provide a description of the power analysis.

6. Was the sample size adequate? Provide a rationale. ____________________

7. What was the sample attrition for this study? ______________________________

8. Was probability or nonprobability sampling used in this study? ______________________________

9. What specific type of sampling method was used in this study? ______________________________

10. Was the sample in this study representative of the target population studied? Provide a rationale. ______________________________

11. Can the findings be generalized? Provide a rationale. ______________________________

12. Where was the setting for this study? ______________________________

    Was the setting natural, partially controlled, or highly controlled? ______________________________

Ågård, Egerod, Tønnesen, and Lomborg (2012) Study

Directions: Review the Ågård et al. (2012) study in Appendix A and answer the following questions.

1. Identify the study population. ______________________________

2. List the sample criteria for this study. ______________________________

3. Identify the sample characteristics for this study. ______________________________

4. What was the sample size? ______________________________

5. Was the sample size adequate? Provide a rationale. ______________________________

6. What was the sample attrition number and rate for this study? ______________________________

7. Was probability or nonprobability sampling used in this study? ______________________________

8. What specific type of sampling method was used in this study? ______________________________

9. Can the findings be generalized? Provide a rationale. ______________________________

10. What were the study settings for the patients' and the partners' interviews? ______________________________

Were the settings natural, partially controlled, or highly controlled? ______________________________

Angélica Martinez

CHAPTER 10

Clarifying Measurement and Data Collection in Quantitative Research

INTRODUCTION

You need to read Chapter 10 and then complete the following exercises. These exercises will assist you in learning key terms and identifying and critically appraising measurement and data collection procedures in published studies. The answers for these exercises are in the Answer Key at the back of the book.

EXERCISE 1: TERMS AND DEFINITIONS

Measurement Concepts and Methods

Directions: Match each term below with its correct definition. Each term is used only once and all terms are defined.

Terms

a. Direct measures
b. Indirect measures
c. Interval level measurement
d. Interview
e. Likert scale
f. Measurement error
g. Nominal level measurement
h. Ordinal level measurement
i. Random measurement error
j. Rating scales
k. Ratio level measurement
l. Structured observational measurement
m. Systematic measurement error
n. True measure or score
o. Visual analog scale

Definitions

g 1. Lowest level of measurement when data can be organized into categories that are exclusive and exhaustive, but the categories cannot be rank-ordered.

m 2. Error that occurs consistently in one direction, such as a scale that weighs everyone 2 pounds less than their true weight, that can alter study results, and must be minimized.

i 3. Error that is the difference between the measurement and true value of a variable that is without a pattern.

e 4. A multiple-item scale used to measure perceptions of a phenomenon in a study, such as a 20-item scale used to measure perception of pain with ratings of 1—strongly disagree, 2—disagree, 3—agree, and 4—strongly agree.

j 5. Older scaling technique requiring patients to judge the level of their symptoms, such as a nurse asking patients to identify their level of pain on a scale of 1 to 10.

h 6. Level of measurement with categories that can be rank-ordered, such as levels of functional status—poor functional status, average functional status, and good functional status.

Angela Martinez

o 7. A scale that uses a 100-mm line for a subject to mark that indicates the placement of his or her score.

a 8. Concrete variables (i.e., blood pressure and pulse) involve these types of measures.

d 9. Questions posed orally to a study participant as a way of collecting data.

c 10. Level of measurement with equal intervals, but without an absolute zero.

b 11. Measurement of abstract ideas (i.e., anxiety and stress) involve these types of measures.

n 12. Ideal or perfect measure that does not include error.

f 13. Difference between the true measure and the actual measure.

k 14. Level of measurement with equal intervals and an absolute zero point.

l 15. Measurement method that requires observation of specific elements in a situation.

Reliability, Validity, Accuracy, and Precision in Measurement

Directions: Match each term below with its correct definition. Each term is used only once and all terms are defined.

Terms

a. Accuracy
b. Alternate forms reliability
c. Content validity
d. Evidence of validity from contrasting groups
e. Evidence of validity from convergence
f. Evidence of validity from divergence
g. Internal consistency reliability
h. Interrater reliability
i. Precision
j. Readability level
k. Reliability
l. Test–retest reliability
m. Validity

Definitions

m 1. Determination of how well an instrument or scale reflects the abstract concept being examined.

a 2. Addresses the extent to which the physiological instrument or equipment measures what it is supposed to in a study and is comparable to validity for scales.

k 3. Concerned with the consistency of a measurement method.

e 4. Type of validity where two scales measuring the sample concept like depression are administered to a group at the same time and the subjects' scores on the scales should be positively correlated.

g 5. Reliability testing used primarily with multi-item scales where each item on the scale is correlated with all of the other items to determine the consistency of the scale in measuring a concept.

l 6. Repeated measures with a scale or instrument to determine the consistency or stability of the instrument in measuring a concept.

j 7. Conducted to determine the participants' ability to read and comprehend the items on an instrument.

d 8. Type of validity where an instrument or scale is given to two groups that are expected to have opposite or contrasting scores, where one group scores high on the scale and another scores low.

c 9. Examines the extent to which a measurement method includes all of the major elements relevant to the concept being measured; review of scales by experts adds to this type of validity.

i 10. Degree of consistency or reproducibility of the measurements made with physiological instruments or equipment; comparable to reliability for scales.

f 11. Type of validity where two scales that measure opposite concepts, such as hope and hopelessness, administered to subjects at the same time should result in negatively correlated scores on the scales.

h 12. Comparison of two observers or judges in a study to determine their equivalence in making observations or judging events.

b 13. Type of reliability involving a comparison of two paper-and-pencil instruments to determine their equivalence in measuring a concept.

Data Collection

Directions: Match each term below with its correct definition. Each term is used only once and all terms are defined.

Terms

a. Administrative data
b. Data collection
c. Data collection form
d. Data collection plan
e. Primary data
f. Secondary data

Definitions

_____ 1. Detailed plan of how the study will be implemented that is specific to the study being conducted and requires consideration of the common elements of the research process.

_____ 2. The actual process of selecting subjects and gathering data from these subjects by the researchers.

_____ 3. Template developed or modified by the researcher that is used for recording data.

_____ 4. Data that are collected for a particular study.

_____ 5. Data collected for reasons other than research, such as the data collected within clinical agencies.

_____ 6. Data collected from previous research, stored in a database, and later used in other studies.

EXERCISE 2: LINKING IDEAS

Directions: Fill in the blanks in this section with the appropriate word(s)/response(s).

1. A fasting blood sugar is an example of what level of measurement? Ratio level measurment

2. A reliability value of at least 0.8 is usually considered a strong coefficient for a scale that has documented reliability and has been used in several studies.

3. In nominal measurement, the categories must be exclusive and exhaustive.

4. Ordinal data have unequal intervals, whereas interval data have ~~eg~~ equal intervals.

Angelica Martinez

5. A questionnaire is a self-report form designed to elict information through written, verbal, or electronic responses of the subject.

6. Temperature is an example of interval level of measurement.

7. The Cronbach's alpha coefficient for perfect reliability is 1.00.

8. A newly developed multi-item Likert scale to measure hope was administered to a group of patients with depression and had a Cronbach alpha of 0.70. Was the scale **reliable** or **unreliable** in this study? reliable

9. The common analysis conducted to determine homogeneity reliability of a scale that has measurement at least at the interval level is the ~~Crohn~~ Cronbach's ~~alpa~~ alpha.

10. If a study's measurement is not reliable, (**it is** or **it is not**) valid. *(Circle correct answer.)* [circled: it is not]

11. When critically appraising the measurement section of a study, you need to check for information about the reliability and reliability of a scale.

12. A(n) unstructured interview includes broad questions and is commonly used in qualitative research.

13. A(n) Structured interview is designed with specific questions to be asked by the researcher and is similar to a questionnaire, which are commonly used in quantitative studies.

14. Which has a higher response rate: mailed questionnaire or personal interview? personal interview

15. FACES scale used to measure perception of pain in children is a(n) rating scale.

16. A scale 100-mm long used to measure anxiety is a(n) visual analog scale scale.

17. Describe three situations that might result in error in researchers' measurement of study variables.

   a. ______

   b. ______

   c. ______

Measurement Error

Directions: Match the type of measurement error likely to occur with the measurement methods listed below. You may use the types more than once.

Type of Error

a. Random error
b. Systematic error

Measurement Methods

_____ 1. Community income using a white, middle-class sample.

_____ 2. Severity of cancer at diagnosis in a community, using patients in a county hospital.

_____ 3. Average body weight measured at work at noon.

_____ 4. Blood pressure taken with equipment that consistently measures the blood pressure low.

_____ 5. Scores on drug calculation tests taken in the morning in a classroom.

Levels of Measurement

Directions: Match the level of measurement with the variables or measures listed below. You may use the categories more than once.

Level of Measurement

a. Nominal
b. Ordinal
c. Interval
d. Ratio

Variables

_____ 1. Temperature

_____ 2. Gender

_____ 3. Educational level

_____ 4. Final exam grade of 90%

_____ 5. Type of cancer

_____ 6. Severity of illness level

_____ 7. Score from visual analog scale

_____ 8. Diagnosis of dyslipidemia

_____ 9. Amount of stress measured with a Likert scale

_____ 10. Height

_____ 11. Percentage of weight gain

_____ 12. Hemoglobin level

_____ 13. Pain level ranking

_____ 14. Body mass index (BMI)

_____ 15. Systolic and diastolic blood pressure

_____ 16. Years of work experience

_____ 17. Ethnicity or race

_____ 18. Hospital vs. hospice

_____ 19. Salary ranges

_____ 20. Marital status

Scales

Directions: Identify the type of scale being presented in the following examples.

Type of Scale

a. Likert scale
b. Rating scale
c. Visual analog scale

Examples

_____ 1. I am satisfied with my nursing education: Agree Neutral Disagree

_____ 2. No Pain |____| Most Severe Pain Possible

_____ 3. On a scale of 1 to 10, how much stress are you feeling?

Sensitivity and Specificity

Directions: Answer the questions in this section.

1. Complete the three boxes in the table below.

Diagnostic test results	Disease present	Disease not present or absent
Positive test	*a* (true positive)	
Negative test		

2. What is the formula for sensitivity?______________________________

3. What is the formula for specificity?______________________________

Sensitivity and Specificity of Colonoscopy Screening Tests

Diagnostic test results	Disease present	Disease not present or absent	Totals
Positive test	250	55	305
Negative test	50	750	800
Totals	300	805	1105

4. What is the number of false positives for the colonoscopy screening test in the previous table? ______________

5. What is the percentage of false positives for the colonoscopy screening test using the data in the previous table?

____

6. What is the number of false negatives for the colonoscopy screening test? ______________________________

7. What is the percentage of false negatives for the colonoscopy screening test? ______________________________

8. What is the sensitivity of the colonoscopy screening test? ______________________________

9. What is the specificity of the colonoscopy screening test? ______________________________

10. What is the positive likelihood ratio (LR) formula? ______________________________

11. What is the positive LR for the colonoscopy screening test? ______________________________

12. What is the negative LR formula? ______________________________

13. What is the negative LR for the colonoscopy screening test? ______________________________

EXERCISE 3: WEB-BASED INFORMATION AND RESOUCES

Directions: Complete the following questions.

1. Search for and identify the Agency for Healthcare Research and Quality (AHRQ) National Quality Measures Guideline website.

   ____

   Review the resources that are available on this website.

2. Search for a national website that discusses the Center for Epidemiologic Studies Depression Scale (CES-D). Identify this website:

   ____

   Review the materials that are available on the CES-D.

3. There is a CES-D scale to screen children for depression. Locate a website that describes this scale.

   ____

4. Identify a website for the Wong-Baker FACES pain rating scale.______________________________

   ____

5. Knapp, Sole, and Byers (2013) measured stress with the State-Trait Anxiety Inventory (STAI) by Spielberger. Locate a website for this scale and review the relevant information.

   ____

6. The STAI requires purchasing for use. Identify a website where the scale might be purchased. ______________

   ____

EXERCISE 4: CONDUCTING CRITICAL APPRAISALS TO BUILD AN EVIDENCE-BASED PRACTICE

Directions: Review the quantitative research articles in Appendices B and C and answer the following critical appraisal questions in the spaces provided.

Bindler, Bindler, and Daratha (2013) Study

1. In the following table, identify the measurement methods for selected variables in the Bindler et al. (2013) study. Also indicate whether the measurement method is a direct or indirect method of measuring the study variables.

Variable(s)	Measurement method(s)	Direct or indirect measurement method
Insulin resistance (IR)		
Total cholesterol (TC), high-density lipoprotein-cholesterol (HDL-C), and low-density lipoprotein-cholesterol (LDL-C)		
Body mass index (BMI)		
Blood pressure: Systolic blood pressure (SBP) and diastolic blood pressure (DBP)		

2. Identify the precision and accuracy information for the following measurement methods.

Variable(s) and measurement methods	Precision and accuracy information from study
HOMA-IR	
Blood pressure: Cuff, stethoscope, and sphygmomanometer	

3. Critically appraise the quality of the measurement of HOMA-IR and blood pressure measures.

HOMA-IR: ____

____

____

____

SBP and DBP: ______________________________

4. Describe the data collection process for the Bindler et al. (2013) study. ______________________________

5. Critically appraise the quality of the data collection process in the Bindler et al. (2013) study. ______________________________

Knapp, Sole, and Byers (2013) Study

1. Identify the measurement methods for selected variables in the Knapp et al. (2013) study in the following table. Also indicate whether the measurement method is a direct or indirect method of measuring the study variables.

Variable(s)	Measurement method(s)	Direct or indirect measurement method
Stress		
Coping		

2. Identify the reliability and validity of the following measurement methods.

Variable(s) and measurement methods	Reliability and validity information from study
Stress: STAI	
Coping: WAYS	

3. Critically appraise the reliability and validity of the STAI.______________________________

____

____

____

____

____

4. Critically appraise the reliability and the validity of the WAYS. ____________________

5. Describe the data collection process for the Knapp et al. (2013) study. ____________________

6. Critically appraise the quality of the data collection process in the Knapp et al. (2013) study. ____________________

Angelica Martinez

CHAPTER

11 Understanding Statistics in Research

INTRODUCTION

You need to read Chapter 11 and then complete the following exercises. These exercises will assist you in learning key terms and identifying and critically appraising statistical techniques, results, and discussion sections in published studies. The answers to these exercises are in the Answer Key at the back of the book.

EXERCISE 1: TERMS AND DEFINITIONS

Directions: Match each term below with its correct definition. Each term is used only once and all terms are defined.

Terms

a. Alpha
b. Decision theory
c. Descriptive statistics
d. Dependent (paired) groups
e. Effect size
f. Generalization
g. Implications for nursing
h. Independent groups
i. Inferential statistics
j. Outliers
k. Post hoc analysis
l. Power
m. Probability theory
n. Type I error
o. Type II error

Definitions

_o_ 1. Error that occurs with the acceptance of the null hypothesis when it is false.

_c_ 2. Summary statistics that allow researchers to organize data in ways that give meaning and facilitate insight.

_f_ 3. Findings acquired from a specific study that are applied to a target population.

_n_ 4. Error that occurs with the rejection of the null hypothesis when it is true.

_e_ 5. Indicates the degree to which a phenomenon is present in a population, such as the strength of a relationship between two variables, or the degree to which the null hypothesis is false.

_m_ 6. Theory used to explain the extent of a relationship, the likelihood an event will occur in a given situation, or the likelihood that an event can be accurately predicted.

_b_ 7. Theory with the assumption that all of the groups used to test a particular hypothesis are components of the same population relative to the variables under study.

_j_ 8. Subjects or data points with extreme values that seem unlike the rest of the sample.

Angelica Martinez

a 9. Level of significance that is set at the start of a study.

g 10. The meaning of research findings for the body of nursing knowledge, theory, and practice.

l 11. The probability that a statistical test will detect a significant difference or relationship that exists.

d 12. Paired groups where subjects in the control group are matched to the subjects in the experimental group based on selected variables, such as levels of an illness or age.

h 13. Groups selected so the participants are unrelated to the selection of other subjects.

i 14. Statistics designed to address objectives, questions, or hypotheses in studies to allow inference from the study sample to the target population.

k 15. Data analysis after an analysis of variance (ANOVA) to determine differences among three groups.

EXERCISE 2: LINKING IDEAS

Directions: Fill in the blanks with the appropriate word(s)/response(s).

1. List five different types of results obtained from the statistical analyses conducted for quasi-experimental and experimental studies.

   a. significant results that agree with those predicted by the researcher

   b. nonsignificant results

   c. significant results that are opposite from those predicted by researcher

   d. mixed results

   e. unexpected results

2. Identify five major ideas or content areas included in the Discussion section of a research report.

   a. Limitations

   b. Conclusions

   c. Implication for nursing

   d. Reccommendations for further studies

   e. Generalizations of the findings.

3. List three steps that researchers conduct during the data analysis process to determine the results for their study.

   a. Management of missing data

   b. Description of the ~~data~~ sample

   c. Reliability of measurement Methods

Angelica Martinez

4. The purpose of statistical analysis is to examine, reduce and give meaning to the numerical data gathered in a study.

5. List four statistical analysis techniques used to describe the sample.

   a. ____________________

   b. ____________________

   c. ____________________

   d. ____________________

6. Draw and label a normal curve with a mean of 0 and a standard deviation of 1.

7. In a normal distribution of scores, what percent of the scores fall between –1.96 and +1.96 standard deviations of the mean? 95%

8. The most precise level of statistical significance is achieved by conducting a (**one-tailed** or **two-tailed**) level of significance. *(Circle correct answer.)*

9. A Type I error occurs if you say that a therapeutic touch intervention works to relieve acute pain when it does not.

10. The abbreviation for analysis of variance is ANOVA.

11. The measure of central tendency calculated for nominal level data is mode.

12. What does "*n*" represent in a statistical table that includes the results from the experimental and comparison groups in a study? Group Size

13. A distribution of data that is asymmetrical because of outliers is called a(n) Skewed or abnormally distributed curve.

Angelica Martinez

14. A diagram of points placed at their relative scores along a best fit line is called a(n) Scatterplot.

15. Data analysis that is conducted on two variables is called bivariate analysis.

Linking Statistics with Analysis Techniques

Directions: Match each statistic with its appropriate analysis technique. Each statistic is used only once, and all analysis techniques have a statistic included.

Statistics

a. *df*
b. *SD*
c. *r*
d. *ES*
e. *R*
f. *F*
g. χ^2
h. %
i. *t*
j. α

Analysis Techniques

_____ 1. Standard deviation

_____ 2. Regression analysis

_____ 3. Alpha

_____ 4. Pearson product-moment correlation

_____ 5. Analysis of variance

_____ 6. Degrees of freedom

_____ 7. Percentage

_____ 8. Chi-square

_____ 9. Effect size

_____ 10. *t*-test

Linking Levels of Measurement with Analysis Techniques

Directions: Link the appropriate level of measurement for data to be analyzed by each of the following analysis techniques. The levels of measurement can be used more than once. Some of the statistical analyses can be used for two different levels of measurement.

Levels of Measurement for Data

a. Nominal level
b. Ordinal level
c. Interval/ratio level

Statistical Analysis Techniques

_____ 1. *t*-test for independent groups

_____ 2. Chi-square

_____ 3. Mean

_____ 4. Pearson product-moment correlation

_____ 5. Percentages

_____ 6. Median

_____ 7. Regression analysis

_____ 8. Effect size

_____ 9. Standard deviation

_____ 10. Range

_____ 11. Mode

_____ 12. Ungrouped frequencies

_____ 13. Analysis of variance

_____ 14. *t*-test for dependent groups

_____ 15. Grouped frequencies

Statements, Inferences, and Generalizations

Directions: Match the statement category with its example study. Each statement category is used only once.

Statement Categories

a. Decision theory statement
b. Probability theory statement
c. Inference
d. Generalization

Example Studies

_____ 1. The experimental pain assessment tool can be used to successfully assess pain levels in hospitalized patients after many different types of surgery.

_____ 2. This suggests that when stress occurs, disruption in social activity is likely to occur.

_____ 3. No significant differences were found in functional outcomes between the two groups of patients treated with sterile petroleum gauze or sterile nonmedicated gauze.

_____ 4. Because most major risk factors thought to affect mental health did not change, and no adverse changes in sleepiness were observed during the intervention period, it is plausible to argue that the music intervention would not have reduced insomnia reports over longer time periods.

Describing the Sample

Directions: Referring to the table below, answer the questions that follow in the spaces provided.

Nurses (N = 100)	Frequency (f)	Percentage (%)
Age in Years		
18-29	10	10%
30-39	20	20%
40-49	35	35%
50-59	30	30%
60 and greater	5	5%
Nursing Education		
Associate's Degree in Nursing (ADN)	50	50%
Diploma	20	20%
Bachelors' of Science in Nursing (BSN)	30	30%
Nurses' Years of Experience	Mean = 15.5 (*SD* = 2.3)	

1. Which variable contains grouped data? ______________________________

2. What is the mode of "Nursing Education"? ______________________________

3. What is the median "Age Group"? ______________________________

4. What is the standard deviation for the "Nurses' Years of Experience"? ______________________________

5. 95% of the nurses' years of experience are between what years? ______________________________

____

Measures of Central Tendency

Directions: Referring to the results of a 10-item Likert scale with response options of 1-5, printed below, answer the questions in the spaces provided.

mean = 3.42   *SD* = 0.76
median = 3.10   mode = 3.00

1. Which value is the average? ______________________________

2. Which value is the 50th percentile? ______________________________

3. What does the mode represent? ______________________________

4. Using the *SD* value, calculate the range of values ± 1 *SD* from the mean. ______________________________

____

____

____

Name That Statistical Analysis Technique!

Directions: Match the following statistical analysis results with the correct analysis technique. Identify the purpose of each analysis technique and the level of measurement (i.e., nominal, ordinal, interval, or ratio) required for conducting the technique.

Statistical Analysis Results

a. $\chi^2 = 4.61$	$df = 2$	$p = 0.10$
b. $t = 15.631$	$df = 180$	$p = 0.001$
c. $r = -0.315$	$df = 76$	$p < 0.05$
d. $F = 36.71$	$df = 420$	$p < 0.001$

_____ 1. ANOVA

Purpose of analysis: ____________________

Level of measurement of data analyzed with this technique: ____________________

_____ 2. Chi-square

Purpose of analysis: ____________________

Level of measurement of data analyzed with this technique: ____________________

_____ 3. Pearson product-moment correlation

Purpose of analysis: ____________________

Level of measurement of data analyzed with this technique: ____________________

_____ 4. *t*-test

Purpose of analysis: ____________________

Level of measurement of data analyzed with this technique: ____________________

Significance of Results

Directions: In the following statistical findings, indicate whether the results were statistically significant (*) or not statistically significant (NS), assuming a level of significance set at alpha = 0.05. You may use each category more than once.

* = Statistically significant
NS = Not statistically significant

_____	1. $\chi^2 = 1.61$	$df = 2$	$p = 0.10$
_____	2. $t = 15.631$	$df = 180$	$p = 0.001$
_____	3. $r = -0.315$	$df = 76$	$p < 0.05$
_____	4. $F = 1.37$	$df = 25$	$p = 0.23$
_____	5. $R = .576$	$df = 130$	$p = <0.001$

EXERCISE 3: WEB-BASED INFORMATION AND RESOURCES

Directions: Answer the following questions with the appropriate website or relevant information.

1. Search the Elsevier website for your textbook, *Understanding Nursing Research*, 6th edition (http://evolve.elsevier.com/grove/understanding/) and find the following study:

   Farrell, G. A., & Shafiei, T. (2012). Workplace aggression, including bullying in nursing and midwifery: A descriptive survey (the SWAB study). *International Journal of Nursing Studies, 49*(11), 1423-1431.

   a. What descriptive statistics were conducted in this study? ______________________________

   ____

   ____

   ____

   b. What inferential statistic was conducted in this study? ______________________________

   ____

   c. What conclusions were reached in this study? ______________________________

   ____

   ____

   ____

   ____

   ____

   ____

   ____

   ____

   d. What suggestions were made for further research? ______________________________

   ____

   ____

   ____

   ____

   ____

   ____

2. Search the Elsevier website for *Understanding Nursing Research*, 6th edition (http://evolve/elsevier.com/grove/understanding/) and find the following study:

   Aronson, B., Glynn, B., & Squires, T. (2013). Effectiveness of a role-modeling intervention on student nurse simulation competency. *Clinical Simulation in Nursing, 9*(4), e121-e126.

   a. What descriptive statistics were conducted in this study? ____________________

   ____

   ____

   ____

   b. What inferential statistics were conducted in this study and what was the purpose of each? ____________________

   ____

   ____

   ____

   c. What limitations were identified for this study?____________________

   ____

   ____

   ____

   ____

   ____

   ____

3. Wikipedia provides a list of several statistical resources. Identify the Wikipedia website for statistical analysis.

   ____

4. The following workbook can provide you additional information about statistical analysis and assist you in critically appraising the results sections of published studies:

   Grove S. K. (2007). *Statistics for health care research: A practical workbook.* St. Louis, MO: Saunders Elsevier.

   Locate this resource on the amazon.com website.

EXERCISE 4: CONDUCTING CRITICAL APPRAISALS TO BUILD AN EVIDENCE-BASED PRACTICE

Bindler, Bindler, and Daratha (2013)

Directions: Read the Bindler, Bindler, and Daratha (2013) study found in Appendix B and then answer the following questions in the spaces provided.

1. How many groups did this study have, and what were the names of the groups? ________________________

____

____

____

2. For each variable in the table, indicate the level of measurement (i.e., nominal, ordinal, interval, or ratio) and the descriptive analysis technique(s) that were conducted in the Bindler et al. (2013) study.

Demographic and study variables	Level of measurement	Descriptive analysis techniques
Age (months)		
Body mass index (BMI)		
Total cholesterol		
Systolic blood pressure (SBP)		

3. What inferential statistics were conducted in this study and what was the purpose of each? ________________

____

____

____

____

____

____

____

4. What was the mean insulin-resistant (HOMA-IR) value in the study? Did males or females have the highest HOMA-IR value? Were the HOMA-IR values significantly different based on gender? Provide a rationale for your answer.

____

____

____

____

____

____

5. What study variable had the strongest correlation or relationship with HOMA-IR? ______________

____

6. The following result was found on in Table 3 of the Bindler et al. (2013) study:

   $r = .560, p < 0.001$

   a. Is this result statistically significant? ______________________________

   b. Is this result clinically important? Provide a rationale for your answer. ______________

   ____

   ____

   ____

7. What variables were used to predict HOMA-IR in this study? (*Hint*: Review results in Table 4 of the Bindler article.)

____

____

8. "The strongest predictive model included waist circumference ($p = .002$) and triglycerides ($p < .001$) as significant predictors of HOMA-IR, $F(2, 146) = 4.69, p < .001$." (Bindler et al., 2013, p. 23)

   a. Is this result statistically significant? ______________________________

   b. Is this result clinically important? Provide a rationale for your answer. ______________

   ____

   ____

   ____

9. What are the implications for nursing practice? ______________________________

Knapp, Sole, and Byers (2013)

Directions: Read the Knapp, Sole, and Byers (2013) study found in Appendix C and then answer the following questions in the spaces provided.

1. For each variable in the table, indicate the level of measurement (i.e., nominal, ordinal, interval, or ratio) and the descriptive analysis technique(s) that were conducted in the Knapp et al. (2013) study.

Demographic variables	Level of measurement	Descriptive analysis techniques
Relationship to patient		
Gender		
Ethnicity		
Patient age (years)		
Patient days in the SICU		

2. Were the anxiety levels significantly different for the experimental and control groups? Provide a rationale for your answer.

3. Eight different subsets of coping were measured. Were any of these subsets of coping significantly different for the experimental and control groups? (*Hint*: Examine the results in Table 2 of the Knapp article.)

____

4. Table 2 in the Knapp article included the following result:

   Distancing control: $t = -2.030$, $p = .023$

   a. Is this result statistically significant? ______________________

   b. What does this result mean? ______________________

   ____

   ____

   ____

5. Identify some of the limitations of this study. Did these limitations have an effect on the study results?

____

____

____

____

____

____

____

____

6. Did the researchers generalize their findings? Was this appropriate based on this study? ______________

____

____

____

____

____

____

____

____

CHAPTER 12

Critical Appraisal of Quantitative and Qualitative Research for Nursing Practice

INTRODUCTION

You need to read Chapter 12 and then complete the following exercises. These exercises will assist you in understanding the quantitative and qualitative research critical appraisal processes. The answers to these exercises are in the Answer Key at the back of the book.

EXERCISE 1: TERMS AND DEFINITIONS

Directions: Match each term below with its correct definition. Each term is used only once and all terms are defined.

Terms

a. Confirmability
b. Critical appraisal
c. Dependability
d. Referred journals
e. Transferable
f. Credibility

Definitions

_____ 1. Applicability of qualitative findings to other settings with similar participants.

_____ 2. Published collections of articles that have been critically appraised by expert peer reviewers.

_____ 3. Degree of readers' confidence that the findings from a qualitative research report represent the perspectives of the participants.

_____ 4. Documentation of the steps taken in a qualitative study and the decisions made during data analysis.

_____ 5. Examination of the quality of studies to determine the credibility, significance, and meaning of the findings for nursing.

_____ 6. Extent to which other researchers can review the audit trail of a qualitative study and agree that the authors' conclusions are logical.

EXERCISE 2: LINKING IDEAS

Directions: Fill in the blanks with the appropriate word(s).

1. An intellectual research critical appraisal involves careful examination of all aspects of a study to judge the ______________________, ______________________, ______________________, and ______________________ of the study.

2. Identify three important questions that are part of an intellectual research critical appraisal.

   a. ______________________________

   b. ______________________________

   c. ______________________________

3. Identify at least three reasons why you would critically appraise nursing studies.

   a. ______________________________

   b. ______________________________

   c. ______________________________

4. Adherence to ethical standards in nursing involves protecting participants' ______________________ and obtaining ______________________ ______________________ from the participants.

5. In qualitative research, what components do you expect to find in a quality abstract?

   a. ______________________________

   b. ______________________________

   c. ______________________________

   d. ______________________________

Understanding the Levels of Critical Appraisal for Quantitative Studies

Directions: Match the steps of the quantitative research critical appraisal process with the examples provided.

Steps

a. Identification of the steps of the research process in studies
b. Determination of study strengths and weaknesses
c. Evaluating credibility and meaning of study findings

Examples

_____ 1. The study framework does not clearly link to the variables' conceptual definitions.

_____ 2. Is the study feasible to conduct in terms of the money commitment; researchers' expertise; availability of subjects, facility, and equipment; and ethical considerations?

_____ 3. Identify the methods of measurement, such as Pain Perception Scale or laboratory cholesterol values, used in the study.

_____ 4. Do the findings add to the current body of nursing knowledge?

_____ 5. Is the design linked to the sampling method, study instruments, and statistical analyses?

_____ 6. Are the study findings consistent with the findings of previous studies?

_____ 7. Means, standard deviations, and *t*-tests were conducted to analyze the study data.

_____ 8. Was the sampling method identified in the study?

_____ 9. Are the physiological measures used in a study accurate, precise, selective, and sensitive?

_____ 10. To what populations can the findings be generalized?

_____ 11. Did the sample section of the study identify a power analysis?

_____ 12. Do the data analyses address the study purpose and the research objectives, questions, or hypotheses?

_____ 13. Is the sample size adequate to address the study purpose?

_____ 14. Are the study findings ready for use in practice?

_____ 15. The quasi-experimental study design included only an experimental group and lacked a control group for comparison.

_____ 16. Is the treatment clearly described and consistently implemented?

_____ 17. Was the Center for Epidemiologic Studies Depression Scale (DEPA) reliable and valid in a study?

_____ 18. Knapp et al. (2013) used Lazarus and Folkman's Transactional Model of Stress and Coping as the framework for their study.

_____ 19. Knapp et al. (2013) study had a small sample size and several nonsignificant findings that indicate possible Type II error in the study.

_____ 20. Bindler et al. (2013, p. 25) recommended that "Pediatric nurses should always measure weight and height and then calculate BMI and BMI percentile for youth in all settings, being alert for those children and adolescents outside the recommended weight for height parameters."

Understanding the Levels of Critical Appraisal for Qualitative Studies

Directions: Match the steps of the qualitative research critical appraisal process with the examples provided.

Steps

a. Identification of the steps of the research process in studies
b. Determination of study strengths and weaknesses
c. Evaluating credibility and meaning of study findings

Examples

_____ 1. Could the limitations of the study have been prevented?

_____ 2. Was the qualitative approach identified?

_____ 3. Were the steps taken and the decisions made adequately documented?

_____ 4. Do the findings add to the current body of nursing knowledge?

_____ 5. What precautions did the researcher take in case participants became upset?

_____ 6. Are the study findings a credible reflection of reality?

_____ 7. Were the findings linked to specific quotes or observations?

_____ 8. Was network or snowball sampling used to recruit participants?

_____ 9. Were the interviews long enough to gather robust descriptions?

_____ 10. To what other settings might the findings be transferred?

EXERCISE 3: WEB-BASED INFORMATION AND RESOURCES

Directions: Search, locate, and review the websites identified in the following questions.

1. Quality and Safety Education for Nurses (QSEN) Project has defined quality and safety competencies for nursing and proposed the knowledge, skills, and attitudes (KSAs) to be developed in nursing pre-licensure programs for each competency. These KSAs are for students in baccalaureate programs who are seeking to become registered nurses (RNs). Locate the QSEN website for the pre-licensure KSAs.

   ____

2. Identify the six QSEN competency areas for pre-licensure nursing students.

   a. ____

   b. ____

   c. ____

   d. ____

   e. ____

   f. ____

3. Which QSEN competency is the most closely linked to understanding the research process and critically appraising studies?

   ____

4. Which EBP attitude is focused on critical appraisal of studies? ______________________

   ____

5. Which EBP skill is focused on reading, understanding, and evaluating studies? ______________________

   ____

6. The Magnet Recognition Program was developed by the American Nurses Credentialing Center (ANCC) to recognize healthcare agencies for quality patient care, nursing excellence, and innovations in professional nursing, which requires reading, critically appraising, and applying relevant research knowledge in practice. Identify the Magnet Recognition Program website.

    ____

7. Search for and identify the website that lists the clinical agencies that have Magnet status. ________________

    ____

    Review the agencies on this website. Having Magnet status is important when searching for agencies for employment.

EXERCISE 4: CONDUCTING CRITICAL APPRAISALS TO BUILD AN EVIDENCE-BASED PRACTICE

Directions: Read the research articles in Appendices A, B, and C. Conduct the steps of the quantitative research critical appraisal process on two of the studies. Conduct the qualitative research critical appraisal process on one of the studies. Use the quantitative and qualitative critical appraisal guidelines provided in Chapter 12, Critical Appraisal of Quantitative and Qualitative Research for Nursing Practice, in your textbook, *Understanding Nursing Research*, 6th edition.

1. Conduct a critical appraisal of the Bindler, Bindler, and Daratha (2013) article using the guidelines outlined in your textbook. Many parts of this study were critically appraised in Chapters 1, 2, and 4 through 11 of this study guide.

    a. Identify the steps of the research process in this descriptive correlational study.

    b. Determine the strengths and weaknesses of the steps in the study.

    c. Evaluate the credibility and meaning of the findings for nursing.

2. Conduct a critical appraisal of the Knapp, Sole, and Byers (2013) article using the guidelines outlined in your textbook, *Understanding Nursing Research*, 6th edition. Many parts of this study were critically appraised in Chapters 1, 2, and 4 through 11 of this study guide.

    a. Identify the steps of the research process in this quasi-experimental study.

    b. Determine the strengths and weaknesses of the steps in the study.

    c. Evaluate the credibility and meaning of the findings for nursing.

3. Conduct a critical appraisal of the Ågård, Egerod, Tønnesen, and Lomborg (2012) article using the qualitative critical appraisal guidelines outlined in Chapter 12 of your textbook, *Understanding Nursing Research*, 6th edition. Many parts of this study were critically appraised in Chapters 1, 3 through 7, and 9 of this study guide.

    a. Identify the steps of the research process in the study.

    b. Determine the strengths and weaknesses of this study.

    c. Evaluate the credibility and meaning of the findings for nursing.

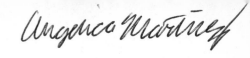

CHAPTER 13

Building an Evidence-Based Nursing Practice

INTRODUCTION

You need to read Chapter 13 and then complete the following exercises. These exercises will assist you in understanding the process of developing an evidence-based practice in nursing. The answers to these exercises are in the Answer Key at the back of the book.

EXERCISE 1: TERMS AND DEFINITIONS

Directions: Match each term with its correct definition. Each term is used only once and all terms are defined.

Terms

a. Algorithms
b. Best research evidence
c. Evidence-based practice
d. Evidence-based practice centers
e. Evidence-based practice guidelines
f. Grove Model for Implementing Evidence-Based Guidelines in Practice
g. Iowa Model of Evidence-Based Practice
h. Meta-analysis
i. Meta-synthesis
j. Mixed-methods systematic review
k. PICOS format
l. Stetler Model of Research Utilization to Facilitate Evidence-Based Practice
m. Systematic review
n. Translation research

Definitions

m 1. A structured, comprehensive synthesis of quantitative studies in a particular healthcare area to determine the best research evidence available for expert clinicians to use to promote evidence-based practice.

k 2. A format for initiating a research synthesis related to a clinical question that includes the following elements: population of interest, intervention needed for practice, comparison of interventions to determine best practice, outcomes needed for practice, and study designs.

h 3. A process of statistically pooling the results from previous studies into a single quantitative analysis that provides a high level of evidence for an intervention's efficacy.

b 4. Highest quality research knowledge produced by the conduct and synthesis of numerous high-quality studies in a health-related area.

Angelica Martinez

e 5. Patient care guidelines that are based on synthesized research findings from systematic reviews, meta-analyses, and extensive clinical trials; supported by consensus from recognized national experts; and affirmed by outcomes obtained by clinicians.

j 6. A process that includes the identification, analysis, and synthesis of research findings from independent quantitative and qualitative studies to determine the current knowledge (what is known and not known) in a particular area.

l 7. This is a comprehensive framework to enhance the use of research findings by nurses that includes the phases of preparation, validation, comparative evaluation/decision making, translation/application, and evaluation.

f 8. Model developed by one of the authors of your textbook, *Understanding Nursing Research*, 6th edition, to promote the use of evidence-based guidelines in practice.

d 9. Centers designated by the Agency for Healthcare Research and Quality for the development of research in designated areas and the translation of the evidence-based research findings into clinical practice.

i 10. A process and product of systematically reviewing, compiling, and integrating qualitative study findings to expand understanding and develop a unique interpretation of the findings in a selected area.

g 11. A model developed by Titler and colleagues in 1994 and revised in 2001 that provides direction for the development of evidence-based practice in a clinical agency.

c 12. A practice that involves the conscientious integration of best research evidence with clinical expertise and patient values and needs in the delivery of quality, cost-effective health care.

a 13. Clinical decision-making trees or figures nurses use when implementing research evidence in practice.

n 14. New and evolving type of research that is defined by the National Institutes of Health (NIH) as a methodology for promoting basic scientific discoveries into practical applications.

EXERCISE 2: LINKING IDEAS

Directions: Fill in the blanks with the appropriate word(s)/response(s).

1. List three reasons nursing needs to develop an evidence-based practice.

   a. Improves quality of care

   b. Decreases cost of care

   c. Increases pt satisfaction with care

2. Identify three sources you might access to keep current with the research literature.

   a. Reading research journals in ~~journals~~ nursing

   b. Attend a professional nursing meetings

   c. Participate in collaborative groups of nurses

Angelica Martinez

3. Identify two barriers or criticisms of evidence-based practice in nursing.

   a. Some healthcare agencies and administiators do not provide resources to implement EBP.

   b. Lack of research evidence available regarding effectiveness of many nursing interventions

4. Identify two reasons why nursing lacks the research evidence needed for implementing an evidence-based practice.

   a. Need for additional studies to determine effcetivness in interventions.

   b. Need for more replication studies to strengthen knowledge

5. Identify and describe three ways that research findings might be implemented in nursing practice that were discussed in Stetler's Model of Research Utilization to Facilitate Evidence-Based Practice.

   a. Immediate Use

   Description: Using research-based ~~intre~~ intervention exactly as it was developed

   b. Reinvention

   Description: When research intervention is modified to meet needs of nurses at agency.

   c. Cognitive Change

   Description: ~~Cognitive Cha~~ when nurses use research findings and incorporate with their knowledge bases and use knowledge to defend a point

6. Identify three sources of summaries of nursing research knowledge.

   a. National Clearinghouse Guildline

   b. Cochrane Library

   c. The National Institute for Health and Clinical Excellnce

7. Identify the five phases of the Stetler Model of Research Utilization to Facilitate Evidence-Based Practice.

   a. Phase I - Preperation

   b. Phase II - Validation

   c. Phase III - Comparitive Evaluation / Decision making

   d. Phase IV - Translation / Application

   e. Phase V - Evaluation

8. The comparative evaluation phase of Stetler's Model includes four parts: substantiating evidence, fit of the setting, feasibility, and current practice.

Angelica Martinez

9. Identify the three options of the decision-making phase of Stetler's Model.

   a. Use research evidence in practice now.

   b. Consider using research knowledge in practice

   c. Do not use research knowledge in practice

10. The National Clearinghouse Guidelines (NCG) website was developed by the Agency for Healthcare Research and quality.

11. The NCG is maintained by a partnership with which two organizations?

    a. American Medical Association (AMA)

    b. American Association of Health Plans (AAHP)

12. In 1997, the Agency for Healthcare Research and Quality established 12 Evidence-Based Practice Centers of Excellence to promote the conduct of research and the development of evidence-based guidelines for practice.

13. NIH is developing funding awards for translational research to improve the Use of evidence in practice.

Application of the Phases of Stetler's Model

Directions: Match the phase in Stetler's Model with the appropriate description and/or example.

Phase

a. Comparative evaluation/decision making
b. Evaluation
c. Preparation
d. Translation/application
e. Validation

Descriptions

_____ 1. The phase in which nurses evaluate the feasibility of using the Braden Scale to prevent pressure ulcers in their clinical agency.

_____ 2. The phase in which nurses develop a formal protocol for treatment of stage IV pressure ulcers in older adults.

_____ 3. The first awareness of the existence of an exercise program for severely disabled children obtained from attending a research conference and reading the study and similar studies in research journals.

_____ 4. Research knowledge about prevention of hospitalized infections is synthesized and evaluated using specific criteria.

_____ 5. The incidence of hospital-acquired infections is examined following the implementation of a new protocol to prevent infections.

Understanding Research Syntheses

Directions: Match the particular type of research synthesis with the appropriate strategies used to conduct these syntheses. Some of the answers include more than one type of research synthesis.

Types of Research Synthesis

a. Systematic review
b. Meta-analysis
c. Meta-synthesis
d. Mixed-methods systematic review

Synthesis Strategies

_____ 1. Research synthesis that involves the statistical pooling of the results from previous studies into a single quantitative analysis that provides one of the highest levels of evidence about the effectiveness of music in promoting rest in an ICU.

_____ 2. Review that includes syntheses of a variety of quantitative and qualitative study designs to determine the current knowledge about medication administration technologies and patient safety.

_____ 3. The systematic compiling and integration of the results from qualitative studies to expand understanding and develop a unique interpretation of study findings to promote an understanding of women's experiences related to losing a child.

_____ 4. A structured, comprehensive synthesis of the research literature to determine the best research evidence available to address a healthcare question, such as the best interventions to promote weight loss in adults. This synthesis might include meta-analysis and other types of research synthesis.

_____ 5. Grey literature should be included in which types of research syntheses?

_____ 6. A preferred reporting statement called PRISMA has been developed to promote consistency and quality in the development of these two types of research syntheses.

_____ 7. Meta-summary is the summarizing of findings across qualitative reports to identify knowledge in a selected area, and this summary is part of this research synthesis.

_____ 8. The PICOS format (**P**opulation, **I**ntervention, **C**omparison, **O**utcomes, and **S**tudy designs) is used to generate a clinical question to direct these types of research synthesis.

_____ 9. A funnel plot might be developed to assess for biases in a group of studies when conducting this type of research synthesis.

_____ 10. The reports from this type of qualitative synthesis might be presented in different formats based on the knowledge developed and the perspective of the authors.

_____ 11. Multilevel synthesis and parallel synthesis are two different approaches that might be used in conducting this type of research synthesis.

_____ 12. Ancestry searches use citations in relevant studies to identify additional studies. Which of these research syntheses use ancestry searches?

_____ 13. One type of research synthesis might use only RCTs and meta-analyses as sources.

_____ 14. This type of research synthesis often includes calculations of risk ratios, odds ratios, and risk differences to determine the effect of an intervention when the outcomes are dichotomous data.

_____ 15. Usually only qualitative studies are included as sources in this type of research synthesis.

Agency's Readiness for Evidence-Based Practice (EBP)

Directions: Think about the clinical agency in which you are currently doing your clinical hours. Provide responses to the following questions and discuss them in class or on your class discussion board.

1. Are the agency's policies, protocols, algorithms, and guidelines based on research? Provide a rationale for your answer.

   ____

   ____

2. If you answered "no" to the previous question, what is the basis of the policies, protocols, algorithms, or guidelines of your agency?

   ____

   ____

3. Who are the individuals identified for promoting EBP changes in this agency? (Record the job titles of those involved.)

   ____

   ____

4. Does the agency provide access to research publications for nurses? If so, provide some examples of these publications.

   ____

   ____

5. Does the agency have the goal of EBP? ______________________________

   ____

6. Is the agency seeking Magnet status? What is the link of EBP to Magnet status? ______________

   ____

   ____

   ____

EXERCISE 3: WEB-BASED INFORMATION AND RESOURCES

Directions: Fill in the blanks below with the appropriate responses.

1. The Agency for Healthcare Research and Quality (AHRQ) National Guideline Clearinghouse at http://www.guidelines.gov provides numerous guidelines to manage nursing problems. On this website, identify where you can search for evidence-based guidelines.

   ____

2. At the http://www.guidelines.gov website, search for EBP guidelines on fall prevention in the elderly. Identify the web address.

____

3. The Oncology Nursing Society website (http://ons.org) has a "Practice Resource" section that includes "Putting Research Evidence into Practice (PEP)." Find this site and locate the EBP guidelines for managing anxiety in patients with cancer.

____

4. Cochrane Nursing Care Field (CNCF) is part of the Cochrane Collaboration and can be found at http://cncf.cochrane.org/. Using that website, identify the site for the Cochrane Reviews in Nursing.

____

5. Locate the Nursing Reference Center (NRC) website. Identify the location for the "Patient Education Reference Center" on this site.

____

6. Locate the U.S. Preventive Services Task Force: Recommendations for Adults website. ____________________

____

7. Locate the following article published by the *Journal of American Medical Association* (JAMA) on the revised guidelines for hypertension:

   James, P. A., Oparil, S., Carter, B. L., Cushman, W. C., Dennison-Himmelfarb, C., Handler, J. et al. (2014). 2014 Evidence-based guideline for the management of high blood pressure in adults: Report from the Panel Members Appointed to the Eighth Joint National Committee (JNC 8). *JAMA, 311*(5), 507-520.

   Where did you locate this source? ____

8. Search for the *Healthy People 2020* website. Identify the location of this website: ____________________

____

9. Identify the website for Genomics that is a new topic for *Healthy People 2020* website: ____________________

____

EXERCISE 4: CONDUCTING CRITICAL APPRAISALS TO BUILD AN EVIDENCE-BASED PRACTICE

Directions: Read and critically appraise the systematic review conducted by Choi and Hector (2012) that focused on the effectiveness of intervention programs in preventing patient falls:

> Choi, M., & Hector M. (2012). Effectiveness of intervention programs in preventing falls: A systematic review of recent 10 years and meta-analysis. *JAMDA, 13*(2), 188.e13–188.e21.

The reference for this study is provided below, and you can search your university library to obtain the study. The critical appraisal was guided by the questions presented in Table 13-2 in Chapter 13 of your textbook, *Understanding Nursing Research*, 6th edition. Your textbook also provides a more detailed critical appraisal of this article.

1. What was the objective of the systematic review, and was it clearly presented? ______

2. Was this systematic review guided by the PICOS format? Provide a rationale for your answer. ______

3. Was the search of the research literature rigorous and clearly described? Provide a rationale to support your answer.

4. How many studies were selected for review? What was the final number of studies selected for the systematic review? Is a detailed discussion and flow chart provided to document the selection process for the studies to be included in the synthesis?

5. How was the quality of the 17 studies assessed? ______

6. Was a meta-analysis conducted as part of this systematic review? ______________________________

7. How did the authors examine the studies for publication bias? Did publication bias exist? ______________________________

____

____

____

8. What was the main conclusion of this systematic review about the effectiveness of fall-prevention programs?

____

____

____

____

____

GOING BEYOND

1. Conduct a project to promote evidence-based practice in a selected area of your practice. Use the following steps as a guide.
   a. Identify a clinical problem using the PICOS format that might be improved by using research knowledge in practice.
   b. Locate and review the research syntheses and studies in this problem area.
   c. Summarize what is known and not known regarding this problem.
   d. Select a model or theory to direct your use of research evidence in practice, such as the Stetler's Model of Research Utilization to Facilitate Evidence-Based Practice, or the Iowa Model of Evidence-Based Practice.
   e. Assess your agency's readiness to make the change.
   f. Communicate the evidence-based change proposed to the nursing personnel, other health professionals, and administration.
   g. Support those persons involved in making the evidence-based change in practice.
   h. Implement the evidence-based change by developing a protocol, algorithm, or policy to be used in practice.
   i. Develop evaluation strategies to determine the effect or outcomes of the evidence-based change on patient, provider, and agency.
   j. Evaluate over time to determine whether the evidence-based change should be continued. You might also extend the change to additional units or clinical agencies.
2. Use the Grove Model for Implementing Evidence-Based Guidelines to implement an evidence-based guideline from the Agency for Healthcare Research and Quality website in your practice.

CHAPTER 14

Introduction to Outcomes Research

INTRODUCTION

You need to read Chapter 14 and then complete the following exercises. These exercises will assist you in learning relevant terms and in reading and comprehending published outcomes studies. The answers for these exercises are in the Answer Key at the back of the book.

EXERCISE 1: TERMS AND DEFINITIONS

Directions: Match each term below with its correct definition. Each term is used only once and all terms are defined.

Terms

a. Administrative databases
b. Clinical databases
c. Distal outcome
d. Nurses' roles in outcomes
e. Nursing care report card
f. Nursing-sensitive patient outcomes
g. Outcomes research
h. Patient health outcomes
i. Proximal outcome
j. Quality of care
k. Standard of care
l. Structures of care

Definitions

_____ 1. These outcomes are influenced by nursing care decisions and actions.

_____ 2. These outcomes are clearly interwoven into the entire care context.

_____ 3. An established field of health research that focuses on the end results of patient care.

_____ 4. Databases that are created by insurance companies, government agencies, and others not directly involved in providing patient care

_____ 5. Have three subcomponents that include nurses' independent role, nurses' dependent role, and nurses' interdependent role.

_____ 6. An outcome that is close to the delivery of care.

_____ 7. This includes a group of indicators that could facilitate the benchmarking, or setting of a desired standard, that would allow comparisons of hospitals in terms of their nursing care quality.

_____ 8. The elements of organization and administration, as well as provider and patient characteristics, that guide the processes of care.

_____ 9. A norm on which quality of care is judged such as clinical guidelines, critical paths, and care maps.

Angelica Martinez

_____ 10. An outcome that is removed from the care or a service received and might be more influenced by external (nontreatment) factors.

_____ 11. The degree to which health services for individuals and populations increase the likelihood of desired health outcomes and are consistent with current professional knowledge.

_____ 12. Databases that are created by providers such as hospitals, clinics, and healthcare professionals.

EXERCISE 2: LINKING IDEAS

Key Ideas

Directions: Fill in the blanks in this section with the appropriate word(s)/ response(s).

1. A major theory dominating outcomes research was developed by Donabedian.

2. Donabedian's cube (see Figure 14-1 in your textbook, *Understanding Nursing Research*, 6th edition) included which three aspects of health?

   a. Physical psychological function
   b. Psychological function
   c. Social function

3. Donabedian identified three foci of evaluation in appraising quality. Identify these three foci and provide an example of each.

   a. Structure: hospitals
   b. process: The care that is provided or practice style
   c. Outcomes: end results of care

4. Loegering, Reiter, and Gambone (1994) modified Donabedian's Model (see Figure 14-2 in your textbook) to include three types of care: care by practioners and other providers, care recieved by community, and care implemented by pt.

5. Nursing Role Effectiveness Model (see Figure 14-3 in your textbook) provided a framework for conceptualizing nursing - sensitive outcomes.

6. Nurses' independent role functions include assessment, ~~diagnoses~~ nursing diagnoses, nurse - initiated interventions, and follow-up care.

7. Nurses' interdependent role functions include such actions as communication, case management, coordination of care, continuity, monitoring, and reporting.

8. To evaluate an outcome as defined by Donabedian, the identified outcomes must be clearly linked to the process of care that caused the outcome.

Angelica Martinez

9. List three examples of standards of care.

   a. Clinical Guidelines

   b. critical paths

   c. care maps

10. The Agency for Healthcare Research and Quality (AHRQ) website is a valuable source of information about outcomes research including funding opportunities and results of recently completed research, nursing research

11. Are (**heterogeneous** or **homogeneous**) samples preferred in outcome studies? *(Circle correct answer.)* [circled: heterogeneous]

12. From an outcomes research perspective, identify three questions nurse researchers might address in conducting outcomes studies.

    a. What are the end results?

    b. What effect does nursing care have on end results?

    c. What are nursing acts that have no effect on outcomes?

13. What are two types of databases that are important sources of data for outcomes studies?

    a. Clinical

    b. Administrative

14. Statistical methods for outcomes studies focus on analysis of Change and improvement.

15. What are the three major questions used for critically appraising outcomes studies?

    a. Are the results valid?

    b. What are the results?

    c. How can I apply the results to pt care?

Outcomes Research Methodologies

Directions: Match each methodology below with its correct description. Each methodology is used only once and all methodologies are described.

Methodologies

a. Population-based studies
b. Prospective cohort study
c. Retrospective cohort study
d. Secondary analysis
e. Standardized mortality ratio (SMR)

Descriptions

C 1. An epidemiological study in which the researcher identifies a group of people who have experienced a particular event for investigation, such as an infection following a surgical procedure.

Angelica Martinez

e 2. The observed number of deaths are divided by the expected number of deaths and multiplied by 100.

a 3. Studies conducted within the context of the patients' community rather than the context of the medical system, such as the elderly individuals' physical and psychological functional levels in their homes.

b 4. An epidemiological study where researchers identify a group of people who are at risk for experiencing a particular event and then follow them over time to observe whether the event occurs, such as the incidence of health problems in morbidly obese individuals.

d 5. A study that involves any reanalysis of data or information collected by another researcher or organization, including analysis of data sets collected from a variety of sources to create time-series or area-based data sets.

EXERCISE 3: WEB-BASED INFORMATION AND RESOURCES

Directions: Supply the full name for each organization acronym. Then, search the web to find these organizations and identify the website for each that discusses their contribution to outcomes research.

1. AHRQ

   Full name: ______________________________

   Website: ______________________________

2. ANA

   Full name: ______________________________

   Website: ______________________________

3. CALNOC

   Full name: ______________________________

   Website: ______________________________

4. NDNQI

   Full name: ______________________________

   Website: ______________________________

5. NINR

   Full name: ______________________________

   Website: ______________________________

6. NIC

   Full name: ______________________________

   Website: ______________________________

7. NQF

   Full name: ______________________________

   Website: ______________________________

8. ONS

   Full name: ______________________________

   Website: ______________________________

EXERCISE 4: CONDUCTING CRITICAL APPRAISALS TO BUILD AN EVIDENCE-BASED PRACTICE

Directions: Locate and read the Galik and Resnick (2013) research article through your university library. The citation for this article is:

> Galik, E., & Resnick, B. (2013). Psychotropic medication use and association with physical and psychosocial outcomes in nursing home residents. *Journal of Psychiatric and Mental Health Nursing, 20*(3), 244-252.

Answer the following questions related to this study.

1. What type of study is the Galik and Resnick (2013) study? Give a rationale for your answer. ______________________________

2. Two major outcomes (physical and psychosocial) were examined in this study (see study title and purpose). What specific variables were measured for these outcomes?

   Physical outcomes measured were: ______________________________

   Psychosocial outcomes measured were: ______________________________

3. What was the design for this study? ______________________________

4. What was the sample size of this study? Critically appraise the sample size of this study. ______

5. What was the setting for this study? Critically appraise the quality of the setting. ______

6. What steps did the researchers take to ensure the study was ethically implemented? ______

7. What method was used to measure the psychosocial outcome of quality of life? Critically appraise the quality of this instrument.

8. What were the key findings from this study? ______

Answer Key to Study Guide Exercises

CHAPTER 1—INTRODUCTION TO NURSING RESEARCH AND EVIDENCE-BASED PRACTICE

EXERCISE 1: TERMS AND DEFINITIONS

Acquiring Knowledge and Research Methods

1. f
2. g
3. d
4. i
5. m
6. b
7. o
8. e
9. k
10. c
11. h
12. j
13. l
14. n
15. a

Evidence-Based Practice Terms

1. e
2. b
3. a
4. d
5. c

Processes Used to Synthesize Research Evidence

1. d
2. a
3. c
4. b

EXERCISE 2: LINKING IDEAS

How Research Influences Practice

1. Description involves identifying the nature and attributes of nursing phenomena. Descriptive knowledge generated through research can be used to identify what exists in nursing practice, to discover new information, and to classify information of use in the discipline. For example, describing those who are at risk for HIV, identifying the signs and symptoms for making a nursing diagnosis, and describing the incidence and spread of infection in healthcare agencies.
2. Explanation focuses on identifying and clarifying the strength and nature of relationships among variables or concepts relevant for practice. For example, risk for developing pressure ulcers is related to level of mobility and age; as mobility decreases and age increases, pressure ulcer risk increases.
3. Prediction involves estimating the probability of a specific outcome in a given situation. For example, research findings predict that family cardiac history, smoking, high cholesterol, and obesity are linked to an increased incidence of heart disease. With predictive knowledge, nurses can anticipate the effects nursing interventions might have on patients and families; for example, predicting the effects of a long-term exercise program on women with breast cancer.
4. Control is the ability to manipulate a situation to produce the desired outcomes in practice. Therefore, nurses could prescribe certain interventions to help patients and families achieve quality outcomes. For example, you would prescribe the use of warm, not cold, applications for the resolution of normal saline IV infiltrations. Stress reduction exercises might be prescribed as an additional treatment for high blood pressure.

Historical Events Influencing Nursing Research

1. Nightingale
2. *Nursing Research*
3. Sigma Theta Tau
4. You might list any three of the following journals:
   Advances in Nursing Science
   Research in Nursing & Health
   Western Journal of Nursing Research
   Scholarly Inquiry for Nursing Practice
   Applied Nursing Research
   Nursing Science Quarterly
5. integrative reviews of research or summaries of current research knowledge in the areas of nursing practice, nursing care delivery, nursing education, and the nursing profession

6. 1985
7. National Institute for Nursing Research (NINR)
8. conduct, support, and dissemination of information
9. Agency for Health Care Policy and Research (AHCPR)
10. Agency for Healthcare Research and Quality (AHRQ)
11. *Healthy People 2020*
12. outcomes research

Acquiring Knowledge in Nursing

1. You could have identified any of the following ways of acquiring knowledge in nursing. Some possible examples of each way of acquiring nursing knowledge are provided.
   a. Tradition: giving a report on hospitalized patients in a specific way or organizing the care provided to the patients in a specific, structured way
   b. Authority: expert nurses, educators, and authors of articles or books
   c. Borrowing: using knowledge from medicine or psychology in nursing practice
   d. Trial and error: positioning a patient in different ways to reduce his or her discomfort during an intramuscular injection or trying different interventions to help patients sleep at night
   e. Personal experience: obtaining knowledge by being in a clinical agency and providing care to patients and families
   f. Role-modeling: a new graduate in an internship being mentored by an expert nurse who models excellent clinical practice behavior
   g. Intuition: knowing that a patient's condition is deteriorating, but having limited concrete data to support this feeling or hunch
   h. Reasoning: reasoning from the general to the specific or deductive reasoning; reasoning from the specific to the general or inductive reasoning
   i. Research: quantitative, qualitative, and outcomes research methods
2. personal experience
3. a. novice
   b. advanced beginner
   c. competent
   d. proficient
   e. expert
4. Research, empirical, or scientific
5. intuition
6. Traditions
7. Deductive reasoning
8. You might identify any of the following important outcomes examined in outcomes research: (a) patient health status (signs, symptoms, functional status, morbidity, mortality); (b) patient satisfaction; (c) costs related to health care; (d) quality of care; (e) quality of care provider; (f) provider satisfaction; and (g) access to care by patients and families.

Linking Research Methods to Types of Research

1.	b	6.	a
2.	b	7.	a
3.	a	8.	a
4.	b	9.	b
5.	a		

Determining the Strength of Levels of Research Evidence

Rank order of the levels of research evidence is 4, 1, 3, 2, 6, 5.

Nurses' Roles in Research

1.	a and/or b	6.	b and/or c
2.	d and/or e	7.	d and e
3.	a, b, c, d, and e	8.	b and/or c
4.	d and/or e	9.	e
5.	b and/or c	10.	d and e

EXERCISE 3: WEB-BASED INFORMATION AND RESOURCES

1. "The mission for the National Institute of Nursing Research (NINR) is to promote and improve the health of individuals, families, communities, and populations. The Institute supports and conducts clinical and basic research and research training on health and illness across the lifespan to build the scientific foundation for clinical practice, prevent disease and disability, manage and eliminate symptoms caused by illness, and improve palliative and end-of-life care." (NINR website: http://www.ninr.nih.gov/aboutninr/ninr-mission-and-strategic-plan)
2. http://www.guidelines.gov
3. http://www.nhlbi.nih.gov/guidelines/hypertension/
4. http://www.healthypeople.gov/2020/
5. http://www.healthypeople.gov/2020/topicsobjectives2020/overview.aspx?topicid=2
6. http://qsen.org/competencies/pre-licensure-ksas/
7. Evidence-Based Practice (EBP) Competency: "Integrate best current evidence with clinical expertise and patient/family preferences and values for delivery of optimal health care." This website also includes the knowledge, skills, and attitudes (KSAs) for the EBP competency.

EXERCISE 4: CONDUCTING CRITICAL APPRAISALS TO BUILD AN EVIDENCE-BASED PRACTICE

Research Methods

1. b
2. c
3. c

Researchers' Credentials

1. The positions of these authors indicate that they have sufficient research and clinical expertise to conduct this study. However, the article does not include the educational credentials for the authors. Ågård works in the Department of Anesthesiology and Intensive Care and the focus of the study is on convalescence of ICU survivors. Limited information is available on this author on the Internet. Dr. Egerod is a clinical professor at the University Hospitals Center for Nursing and Care Research and is an associate professor at Copenhagen University. Dr. Egerod has previous qualitative research publications and clinical expertise in public health and patient safety. Tønnesen is a clinical professor in the Department of Anesthesiology and Intensive Care with previous research publications in the areas of immunology and critical illnesses. An Internet search of Dr. Lomborg identified that she has a PhD in Nursing and is noted for her grounded theory research expertise and clinical experience in care for hospitalized patients with severe respiratory diseases. The study was supported by grants from seven different foundations, organizations, and clinical facilities such as "the Health Insurance Foundation, the Danish Nurses' Origination, Aarhus University Hospital" (Ågård et al., 2012, p. 112). The grant support indicates that the study was reviewed by a variety of experts who chose to financially support the research. These authors have the research and clinical expertise to conduct this study, but the article might have provided information on their educational credentials.
2. Ross Bindler is a PharmD Candidate and the research is probably a requirement related to his doctorate program. Ruth Bindler and Kenn Daratha are both PhD-prepared faculty for the College of Nursing at Washington State University. The PhD indicates these individuals have research expertise and universities require conducting and publishing research as part of the role of a faculty member. Searching Bindler's name on the Internet identified her clinical expertise as pediatrics and she has co-authored several editions of a pediatric nursing textbook. Searching Daratha's name on the Internet identified that he has expertise in statistics and computer science and received an excellence in research award. This study was "supported by an Agriculture and Food Initiative Grant 2007-55215-17909 from the USDA National Institute for Food and Agriculture," indicating the study was reviewed by research experts and financially supported by a federal grant (Bindler et al., 2013, p. 25). Therefore, these authors demonstrate the research, educational, and clinical expertise necessary to conduct this study.
3. Knapp, Sole, and Byers all are PhD-prepared, indicating experience in conducting research. Knapp has two previous publications (Knapp, 2006; Leon & Knapp, 2008) in this area that are identified in the reference list for this article. Knapp, Sole, and Byers are all university faculty members in colleges of nursing. Universities emphasize conducting and publishing research to promote career advancement. A search of Knapp's name on the Internet indicates that she has clinical experience in critical care, family-centered care, and trauma. Search of Sole's name indicates she is a distinguished professor who has been recognized for her research expertise. Byers is a professor of nursing with several funded research projects and publications. These individuals have strong research, educational, and clinical expertise to conduct this study.

Study Titles and Abstracts

1. Title: Bindler et al. (2013) titled their study "Biological correlates and predictors of insulin resistant among early adolescents". This title clearly identifies the study population as adolescents and indicates the type of study, correlational quantitative research. The focus of the study is also clearly identified as biological predictors of insulin resistance, which is a significant topic with the increased prevalence of obesity among youth.
2. Abstract: Critical appraisal of the abstract for the Bindler et al. (2013) study indicated that the study problem was clearly identified and significant with the focus on obesity, insulin resistance (IR), and type 2 diabetes in adolescents. The study purpose, sample size, key study findings, and implications for nursing were concisely presented. The abstract was very brief and would have been strengthened by identification of the study framework and design.

Critical Appraisal of the Titles and Abstracts of Studies on Research Course Discussion Board

Put your critical appraisals of the titles and abstracts for the Ågård et al. (2012) and Knapp et al. (2013) studies on the discussion board for your research course and review the comments of other students. Clarify any questions with your faculty.

CHAPTER 2—INTRODUCTION TO QUANTITATIVE RESEARCH

EXERCISE 1: TERMS AND DEFINITIONS

1. m
2. s
3. a
4. d
5. r
6. c
7. i
8. l
9. q
10. k
11. n
12. o
13. f
14. t
15. h
16. g
17. e
18. j
19. p
20. b

EXERCISE 2: LINKING IDEAS

Control in Quantitative Research

1. highly controlled
2. quasi-experimental and experimental
3. descriptive and correlational
4. experimental
5. nonrandom or nonprobability; random or probability
6. natural
7. highly controlled
8. experimental
9. partially controlled

Steps of the Research Process

1. problem-solving; nursing
2. Step 1: Research problem and purpose
   Step 2: Literature review
   Step 3: Study framework
   Step 4: Research objectives, questions, or hypotheses
   Step 5: Study variables
   Step 6: Research design
   Step 7: Population and sample
   Step 8: Methods of measurement
   Step 9: Data collection
   Step 10: Data analysis
   Step 11: Research outcomes; and you might have also included communication of findings and use of findings in practice.
3. statements taken for granted or considered true, even though they have not been scientifically tested
4. You could identify any of the following assumptions or other assumptions you have noted in a research report.
   a. People want to assume control of their own health problems.
   b. Stress should be avoided.
   c. Health is a priority for most people.
   d. People who live in poor areas feel underserved for health care.
   e. Attitudes can be measured with a scale.
   f. Most measurable attitudes are held strongly enough to direct behavior.
   g. Health professionals view health care in a manner different from that of laypersons.
   h. Human biological and chemical factors show less variation than do cultural and social factors.
   i. People operate on the basis of cognitive information.
   j. Increased knowledge about an event lowers anxiety about the event.
   k. Receipt of health care at home is preferable to receipt of care in an institution.
5. a smaller version of a proposed study that is conducted to develop and/or refine the study methodology, such as the intervention, measurement instruments, or data collection process, to be used in the larger study
6. You could identify any of the following reasons for conducting a pilot study:
   a. To determine whether the proposed study is feasible (e.g., Are the subjects available? Does the researcher have the time and money to conduct the study?)
   b. To develop or refine a research treatment or intervention
   c. To develop a protocol for the implementation of an intervention
   d. To identify problems with the design
   e. To determine whether the sample is representative of the population or whether the sampling technique is effective
   f. To examine the reliability and validity of the research instruments
   g. To develop or refine data collection instruments
   h. To refine the data collection and analysis plan
   i. To give the researcher experience with the subjects, setting, methodology, and methods of measurement
   j. To try out data analysis techniques

Reading Research Reports

1. You could identify any of the following nursing research journals.
   a. *Advances in Nursing Science*
   b. *Applied Nursing Research*
   c. *Biological Research for Nursing*
   d. *Clinical Nursing Research: An International Journal*
   e. *Journal of Nursing Measurement*
   f. *Journal of Nursing Scholarship*

g. *International Journal of Nursing Studies*
h. *International Journal of Nursing Terminologies and Classifications*
i. *Nursing Research*
j. *Nursing Science Quarterly*
k. *Qualitative Nursing Research*
l. *Research in Nursing & Health*
m. *Scholarly Inquiry for Nursing Practice: An International Journal*
n. *Western Journal of Nursing Research*
o. *Worldviews on Evidence-Based Nursing*

2. Look in clinical journals and see which ones have several research articles in each issue. You might have identified any of the following nursing clinical journals:
   a. *Issues in Comprehensive Pediatric Nursing*
   b. *Journal of Transcultural Nursing*
   c. *Heart & Lung: Journal of Acute and Critical Care*
   d. *Journal of Nursing Education*
   e. *Birth*
   f. *Nursing Diagnosis*
   g. *Public Health Nursing*
   h. *The Diabetes Educator*
   i. *Maternal-Child Nursing Journal*
   j. *Journal of Nursing Education*
   k. *Journal of Pediatric Nursing*
   l. *Archives of Psychiatric Nursing*
3. a. Introduction
   b. Methods
   c. Results
   d. Discussion
4. a. Design
   b. Sample
   c. Setting
   d. Methods of measurement
   e. Data collection process

   The methods section also includes the intervention if that is applicable to the type of study being conducted, such as for quasi-experimental and experimental studies.
5. a. Major findings
   b. Limitations of the study
   c. Conclusions drawn from the findings
   d. Implications of the findings for nursing
   e. Recommendations for further research
6. Introduction
7. theoretical and empirical
8. skimming, comprehending, and analyzing
9. identifying and understanding the steps of the research process
10. determining the value of the research report's content by examining the quality and completeness of the steps of the research process and the links among these steps

Types of Quantitative Research

1. c
2. a
3. b
4. a
5. c
6. d
7. a
8. b
9. c
10. d
11. b
12. a
13. c or d
14. a
15. c
16. a
17. b
18. a
19. a
20. b

EXERCISE 3: WEB-BASED INFORMATION AND RESOURCES

1. Descriptive study. The study title indicates it is a descriptive study. The abstract identifies the design as a descriptive study design.
2. Quasi-experimental study. The study title focuses on the effectiveness of a role-modeling intervention, which indicates either a quasi-experimental or experimental type of study. The study abstract identifies the type of study by stating: "The primary purpose of this quasi-experimental pre-test, post-test study was to assess…" (Aronson et al., 2013, p. e121).
3. Search the NINR website (http://www.ninr.nih.gov/) and identify the section "Research Highlights" to determine the types of research being conducted in nursing. The website is http://www.ninr.nih.gov/researchandfunding/researchhighlights.

EXERCISE 4: CONDUCTING CRITICAL APPRAISALS TO BUILD AN EVIDENCE-BASED PRACTICE

Type of Quantitative or Qualitative Research

1. f
2. b
3. c

Type of Setting

1. a. Ågård et al. (2012) study was conducted in a natural setting. The individual interviews took place in the couples' home or in a quiet room at the hospital. The group interviews were conducted in meeting rooms at one of the hospitals.
2. b. Bindler et al. (2013) study was conducted in partially controlled settings of the schools or at the university campus that were structured to do the assessments of the participating students for the measurement of the biological variables.

3. b. Knapp et al. (2013, p. 53) "study was conducted in the 3-bed SICU at a 617 tertiary university medical center in north central Florida with a level-1 trauma center." The structure of the SICU would be considered a partially controlled setting for a study.

Type of Research Conducted (Applied or Basic)
1. a
2. a
3. a

CHAPTER 3—INTRODUCTION TO QUALITATIVE RESEARCH

EXERCISE 1: TERMS AND DEFINITIONS
1. o
2. n
3. l
4. d
5. i
6. m
7. k
8. f
9. j
10. c
11. e
12. g
13. h
14. a
15. b

Definitions in Your Own Words
1. Observation is gathering data by being in specific environments and situations and using all of your senses to notice and record details.
2. Coding is assigning a label to a key phrase or sentence in a transcript. The codes are synthesized into themes.
3. Researcher-participant relationship is the communication and trust that connects the researcher and the participants and through which data are produced.

EXERCISE 2: LINKING IDEAS

People and Their Contributions to Qualitative Research
1. b
2. e
3. c
4. a
5. d

Qualitative Research Methodology
1. immersed
2. native
3. field notes
4. snowball or network
5. moderator

Approaches to Qualitative Research
1. E
2. P
3. H
4. G
5. E
6. ED
7. P
8. H

EXERCISE 3: WEB-BASED INFORMATION AND RESOURCES
1. Although answers may vary, the table includes commonly found descriptions.

Qualitative	Quantitative
Data: words	Data: numbers
Goal: understanding participant's perspective	Goal: generalization beyond the study
Subjective	Objective
Rigor: truth, credibility	Rigor: reliability, validity, study control, type of design
Evolving methods	Predetermined methods
Fewer subjects—more data from each	More subjects—specific, preset data collected
Researcher influences the method and the data collected	Researcher remains objective

Fry (2011)

Study characteristic	Answer
Country/state in which the study was conducted.	Australia
Identify the qualitative approaches used (phenomenology, grounded theory, exploratory-descriptive qualitative, ethnography, historical)	Ethnography
Identify the human experience or topic of the study.	Emergency nursing practice belief systems
Describe the sample.	10 triage nurses
How were the data collected?	Nonparticipant observation

Harvey et al. (2013)

Study characteristic	Answer
Country/state in which the study was conducted.	United States/ Washington
Identify the qualitative approaches used (phenomenology, grounded theory, exploratory-descriptive qualitative, ethnography, historical)	Phenomenology
Identify the human experience or topic of the study.	Experiences of mothers whose infants underwent complex cardiac surgeries
Describe the sample.	8 mothers
How were the data collected	Journal entries of the mothers

Wallace & Storm (2007)

Study characteristic	Answer
Country in which the study was conducted.	United States/ Connecticut
Identify the qualitative approaches used (phenomenology, grounded theory, exploratory-descriptive qualitative, ethnography, historical)	Grounded theory
Identify the human experience or topic of the study.	Psychosocial and educational needs of men diagnosed with prostate cancer
Describe the sample.	16 men with prostate cancer
How were the data collected?	Focus groups

EXERCISE 4: CONDUCTING CRITICAL APPRAISALS TO BUILD AN EVIDENCE-BASED PRACTICE

1. The purpose of the study was "exploring the challenges facing ICU survivors with cohabiting spouse or partner and explain patients' concerns and coping modalities during the first 12 months post ICU discharge" (Ågård et al., 2012, p.106).
2. The qualitative method used was "qualitative, exploratory, longitudinal" study with grounded theory methods (p. 106). This method is appropriate because the topic had been rarely studied and the aim was to obtain the survivors' perceptions of their concerns and coping methods.
3. a. Number who declined to participate = 1
   b. Number excluded = 3
   c. Exclusion criteria included in this study were: Death within first 3 months after discharge and illness exacerbation
4. Data were collected through interviews with couples at 3 and 12 months postdischarge. The researchers also conducted two focus groups between 3 and 12 months postdischarge.
5. a. Shortest length of stay in ICU = 5 days (Participant #3)
   b. Working prehospitalization and not working posthospitalization = 4 (Participants #3, 7, 9, 12)
   c. Longest stay in total = 232 days (Participant #13 stayed 51 days in ICU, 7 days in hospital, 174 days in rehabilitation.)

6. The researchers found patients who were not concerned about the trauma of their ICU stay and psychological complications. "Their focus was on overcoming everyday physical and functional challenges" (p. 110). The researchers found that instead of posttraumatic stress, the patients had demonstrated resourcefulness.
7. Answers will vary depending on student preference.
8. Ågård et al. (2012) recommended studies exploring patient and family concerns from the perspectives of other rehabilitation specialties. They also recognized the need for additional studies on the challenges of ICU patients during hospitalization and postdischarge and on the role of relatives in the recovery of ICU patients.

CHAPTER 4—EXAMINING ETHICS IN NURSING RESEARCH

EXERCISE 1: TERMS AND DEFINITIONS

1. g
2. a
3. i
4. k
5. j
6. e
7. m
8. c
9. o
10. f
11. d
12. n
13. h
14. b
15. l

EXERCISE 2: LINKING IDEAS

1. a. Disclosure of essential study information to the subject
   b. Comprehension of this information by the subject
   c. Competency of the subject to give consent
   d. Voluntary consent by the subject to participate in the study
2. Essential information in a study consent form:
   a. Introduction of the research activities
   b. Statement of the research purpose
   c. Explanation of study procedures
   d. Description of risks for discomfort and harm
   e. Description of benefits
   f. Disclosure of alternatives
   g. Assurance of anonymity or confidentiality
   h. Offer to answer questions
   i. Option to withdraw
   j. Contact information for the researcher(s)
3. Voluntary
4. diminished autonomy
5. institutional review boards (IRBs)
6. a. Exempt from review
   b. Expedited review
   c. Complete or full review
7. To determine the benefit-risk ratio, you need to assess the benefits and risks of the sampling method, consent process, procedures, and outcomes of the study. The proposed study needs to indicate that informed consent and Health Insurance Portability and Accountability Act (HIPAA) release will be obtained from the subjects and selection and treatment of the subjects during the study will be fair. The type of knowledge generated from the study also needs to be examined to determine how this knowledge will impact the subjects (therapeutic or nontherapeutic) and influence nursing practice. The risks need to be reduced, if possible, and should not cause serious harm to the subjects. The benefits need to be maximized, if possible. If the benefits adequately outweigh the risks for the study, then the benefit-risk ratio usually indicates that the study is ethical to conduct. However, the IRB makes the final decision about whether a study can be conducted in an agency.
8. Exempt from review is the most likely answer, but the type of review is determined by the IRB of the agency where the study is to be conducted.
9. Complete review
10. Possible answers include:
    a. Fabrication of data in the research report
    b. Falsification of data in the research report
    c. Forging of data
    d. Manipulation of the design or methods of a study to obtain the results desired
    e. Selectively retaining or manipulating study data
    f. Manipulation of data analyses to obtain the results desired
    g. Plagiarism of another author and/or researcher's work
    h. Named as an author on a publication when the person did not have direct involvement in the study
11. Office of Research Integrity (ORI)
12. Yes, this is an area of concern in nursing. Articles published in nursing journals have outlined the concerns and actions to be taken to control research misconduct in the discipline (see the References in Chapter 4). Haberman et al. (2010) identified five major categories of research misconduct in nursing studies: protocol violations, consent violations, fabrication and falsification of data, and financial conflicts of interest. Journal editors have expressed concerns about research misconduct and have developed guidelines for managing such problems.
13. Yes. An increasing number of animals are being used by nurse scientists to generate basic research

knowledge for the profession. Most of the animals used in research are mice and rats.

14. Office of Laboratory Animal Welfare (OLAW)
15. American Association for Accreditation of Laboratory Animal Care (AAALAC)

Historical Events, Ethical Codes, and Regulations

1. b	6. a
2. c	7. d
3. d	8. b
4. b	9. a
5. c	10. c

Ethical Principles

1. c	4. b
2. a	5. b or c
3. c	

Federal Regulations Influencing the Conduct of Research

Review Table 4-2 for a summary of these regulations.

1. a	4. b
2. c	5. c
3. a	

Ethics of Published Studies

1. e	4. d
2. c, d	5. a
3. b	6. c

EXERCISE 3: WEB-BASED INFORMATION AND RESOURCES

The following websites provide the location of the information requested for each question in this section. Search these websites and identify relevant information related to the ethical conduct of research.

1. http://www.hhs.gov/ohrp/policy/ohrpregulations.pdf
2. http://www.hhs.gov/ohrp/humansubjects/guidance/belmont.html
3. http://www.accessdata.fda.gov/scripts/cdrh/cfdocs/cfcfr/CFRsearch.cfm?CFRPart=50a
4. http://privacyruleandresearch.nih.gov/
5. http://ori.dhhs.gov/case_summary
6. http://grants.nih.gov/grants/policy/air/researchers_institutions.htm

EXERCISE 4: CONDUCTING CRITICAL APPRAISALS TO BUILD AN EVIDENCE-BASED PRACTICE

1. The Ågård et al. (2012) study was conducted in Denmark, but appears to follow similar ethical guidelines to those in the United States. The study has a separate heading titled "Ethical Considerations." The study had "ethical and legal approval from the National Board of Health and the Danish Data Protection Agency" (p. 106), which seems similar to the institutional review board (IRB) approval in the U.S. The potential participants were invited to participate in the study and were "informed about the study verbally and in writing, the right to withdraw at any time, confidentiality and anonymity and asked to sign a letter of informed consent" (p. 106). This statement indicates that the researchers obtained informed consent from the study participants. This study appears to be ethical, because the risks are minimal and the benefits are strong, resulting in a positive benefit-risk ratio.
2. Bindler et al. (2013) indicated that IRB approval and informed consent were obtained. They reported that "University and school district institutional review board approvals and signed parent permission/student assent were obtained" (p. 21). The participants included middle school students who volunteered to participate in a project called TEAMS. Because the students were underage (diminished autonomy), the permission of the parents was required, as well as the assent of the students for study participation. This study has potential therapeutic benefits for the students since they were provided information about their biological factors (BMI, waist circumference, C-reactive protein, cholesterol values, and blood pressure) to determine if they were predictive of insulin resistance (HOMA-IR). However, the ethics of this study would have been stronger if the researchers had mentioned compliance with the HIPAA regulations.
3. Knapp et al. (2013) clearly covered the ethical aspects of their study. They had a heading titled "Ethical Considerations" and stated "The study was approved by the institutional review boards (IRBs) at the research site and the University of Central Florida. All participants signed an informed consent, and were issued a unique identification number to ensure confidentiality" (p. 53). This study appears to have more benefits than risks and the family members of critically ill trauma patients had a potential to benefit from the EPICS intervention used to reduce their stress and improve coping. The researchers documented the institutional review and informed consent processes in their study, but did not include a discussion of HIPAA compliance.

CHAPTER 5—RESEARCH PROBLEMS, PURPOSES, AND HYPOTHESES

EXERCISE 1: TERMS AND DEFINITIONS

1. d
2. i
3. h
4. g
5. j
6. k
7. f
8. e
9. a
10. c
11. b

Types of Hypotheses

1. h
2. g
3. b
4. e
5. c
6. a
7. d
8. f

EXERCISE 2: LINKING IDEAS

Research Problem and Purpose

1. a. variables or concepts
   b. population
   c. setting
2. You might have identified any of the following or thought of another relevant reason:
   a. has an impact on or is used to guide nursing practice
   b. builds on previous research
   c. promotes theory testing and development
   d. addresses current concerns or priorities in nursing
3. You might have identified any of the following agencies or organizations: National Institute for Nursing Research (NINR), American Nurses Association (ANA), American Association of Critical-Care Nurses (AACN), Oncology Nursing Society (ONS), American Organization of Nurse Executives (AONE), or Agency for Healthcare Research and Quality (AHRQ). You might have identified other nursing and healthcare professional organizations that have research priorities identified online or in publications.
4. a. researchers' expertise, which focuses on educational preparation, research previously conducted, and clinical experiences
   b. financial commitment
   c. availability of subjects, facility, and equipment
   d. study's ethical considerations
5. educational, research or clinical

Understanding Hypotheses

1. b, c, d, g
2. a, c, e, g
3. b, c, e, f
4. a, d, g, h
5. b, d, g, h
6. b, c, d, g
7. a, c, d, g
8. b, c, e, f
9. a, c, e, g
10. b, d, g, h
11. You could state the directional hypothesis in either of the following ways:
    a. Increased age, decreased family support, and decreased health status are related to decreased self-care abilities in nursing home residents.
    b. Decreased age, increased family support, and increased health status are related to increased self-care abilities in nursing home residents.
12. Patients with chronic low-back pain receiving low-back massage have no less perceptions of low-back pain than those patients receiving no massage.

Identifying Types of Study Variables

1. a
2. b
3. c
4. a
5. a or b
6. b
7. b
8. c
9. a
10. c
11. c
12. b
13. a
14. b
15. a

Understanding Study Variables

1. a
2. d
3. f
4. c
5. e
6. b

EXERCISE 3: WEB-BASED INFORMATION AND RESOURCES

1. The website is http://www.csrees.usda.gov/. You can review this website for "Grants" to identify the types of funding provided by the USDA National Institute for Food and Agriculture.
2. The website is http://www.cdc.gov/.
3. The website is http://www.cdc.gov/obesity/childhood/index.html.
4. The website is http://www.cdc.gov/obesity/childhood/solutions.html.
5. a. Research topics are: Cardiac infants; oral motor simulation; feeding; nutrition (See Coker-Bolt et al., 2013, p. 64).
   b. "The purpose of this pilot study was to determine the effects of oral motor stimulation on infants born with complex univentricle anatomy who require surgery shortly after birth" (p. 64).

c. This purpose statement is incomplete since it does not include the dependent variables or outcomes for this study that are length of time to reach full bottle-feeds and length of hospital stay. The purpose does identify the independent variable or intervention of oral motor stimulation and the population studied as infants with complex univentricle anatomy.

EXERCISE 4: CONDUCTING CRITICAL APPRAISALS TO BUILD AN EVIDENCE-BASED PRACTICE

Problem and Purpose

Bindler, Bindler, and Daratha (2013) Study

1. a. Significance of the problem: "Prevalence of obesity is at historic high levels among youth; for example, worldwide, obesity has doubled, and in developed countries, the numbers of youth who are overweight or obese have tripled in the last three decades (Ogden et al., 2006; World Health Organization, 2011)" (Bindler et al., 2013, p. 20).
   b. Background of the problem: "Insulin resistance (IR) is associated with obesity and abnormal glucose metabolism and transport and can lead to a prediabetic state (Lee, Okumura, Davis, Herman, & Gurney, 2006…; Liu et al., 2009; Monzavi et al., 2006). In IR, muscle, fat, and liver cells cannot respond adequately to insulin, and therefore, increased insulin production occurs; high levels of both serum glucose and insulin are present at the same time (National Diabetes Information Clearinghouse, 2008)" (Bindler et al., 2013, p. 20).
   c. Problem statement: "Despite the known relationships between IR and cardiometabolic factors, no study has yet examined the independent effects of these factors on a predictive model of IR among early adolescents" (Bindler et al., 2013, p. 21).
2. Study purpose: "Therefore, the purposes of this study among a group of early adolescents participating in the Teen Eating and Activity Mentoring Schools (TEAMS) study were to describe the anthropometric and laboratory markers of participants and to test the ability of these markers to predict risk of exhibiting IR" (Bindler et al., 2013, p. 21). This purpose clearly focuses the study, includes study variables, identifies the study population, and indicates the type of study—descriptive, predictive correlational study.
3. The problem and purpose are significant because the number of adolescents who are overweight and obese has tripled in the last 30 years in developed countries, which increases their risk for IR and type 2 diabetes later in life (see the Problem discussion in Question 1).
4. Yes, the variables, population, and settings are identified.
   a. This is a descriptive, predictive correlational study. The dependent variable of IR was predicted using the independent variables anthropometric markers (height, weight, waist circumference, body mass index [BMI], and body percentile were calculated) and laboratory markers (total cholesterol, low-density lipoprotein-cholesterol [LDL-C], high-density lipoprotein-cholesterol [HDL-C], triglycerides, C-reactive protein [hsCRP]). Systolic blood pressure (SBP) and diastolic blood pressure (DBP) were also measured but were not clearly identified as variables in the study purpose.
   b. Population: Males and females in early adolescence (students in middle schools).
   c. Settings: Schools and university campus
5. The problem and purpose are feasible because (1) the study was funded by the USDA National Institute of Food and Agriculture; (2) Bindler, Bindler, and Daratha had research, educational, and clinical expertise to conduct this study, as discussed in Chapter 2 of this study guide; (3) adequate subjects were available to participate in the study because the population was early adolescents and the settings were middle schools; (4) school personnel were supportive of the study; (5) arrangements were made to obtain the blood samples needed for the study and to conduct the laboratory analysis of the serum; and (5) the study was ethical and protected the rights of the study participants.

Knapp, Sole, and Byers (2013) Study

1. a. Significance of the problem: "Families of critically ill patients experience stress related to the hospitalization of their family members, and their ability to cope varies. Stress may result in behavioral changes, exhaustion, decreased amount or quality of sleep, poor eating habits, worsening of health problems, and posttraumatic stress disorder (Auerbach et al., 2005; Carter & Clark, 2005; McAdam & Puntillo, 2009…)" (Knapp et al., 2013, p. 51).
   b. Background of the problem: "Nurses play an important role in assisting families to manage stress and cope (Chui & Chan, 2007…). However, this assistance varies greatly among

nurses, making its delivery inconsistent" (Knapp et al., 2013, p. 51).

c. Problem statement: "While needs and stressors of families of critically ill have been researched extensively (Auerbach et al., 2005;... Yang, 2008), no studies have been conducted to determine if a formal educational nursing program was effective in reducing family stress and promoting coping... Other research indicated that involving family members in providing oral care to cardiovascular patients decreased family stress, but the intervention was family involvement, not nursing education" (Knapp et al., 2013, p. 51). This study has three sentences that focus on the problem statement. You might have listed any or all three of these sentences that identify the knowledge that is missing, which led to the conduct of this study.

2. a. "The specific aim [purpose] of this research study was to assess the effectiveness of an evidence-based intervention for critical care nurses to assist families of critically ill trauma patients in reducing their stress and improving their coping skills" (Knapp et al., 2013, p. 52).
   b. The purpose did not clearly identify the evidence-based intervention (independent variable) in this study, which was the EPICS Family Bundle. A study purpose should not predict the outcomes of a study; that is best presented in the study hypothesis. This study purpose did predict the study outcomes as reducing stress and improving coping skills.
   c. The purpose might have been more clearly stated as: The purpose of this study was to determine the effects of the EPICS Family Bundle provided by nurses on the stress and coping skills of family members of critically ill trauma patients.
3. The problem and purpose are significant because millions of critically ill trauma patients are hospitalized each year and their family members experience extensive stress and have coping problems. These family members need support from nurses so their health does not deteriorate and they can continue to be supportive of their critically ill family member.
4. The dependent variables, population, and setting are clearly identified in this study purpose. However, the independent variable or intervention of the study is not included in the study purpose; it is in the study title.
   a. Variables: This is a quasi-experimental study that included an evidence-based intervention that should have been identified as the EPICS Family Bundle, a specialized nursing education program. The dependent or outcome variables included in this study are stress and coping levels.
   b. Population for the study was family members of critically ill trauma patients.
   c. Setting for the study is assumed to be intensive care units since the family members were of critically ill trauma patients.
5. This study was feasible because: (a) the researchers had educational, clinical, and research expertise to conduct this study as detailed in Chapter 2 of this study guide; (b) many family members were available since the setting was a large SICU with many critically ill trauma patients; (3) the study required educational materials and instructors provided within the hospital; and (4) the study appeared ethical since there were potential benefits for the family members and limited potential for risks. The study had IRB approval and all participants signed an informed consent. No specific funding for the study was identified, but the researchers did seem to have the support of the hospital.

Ågård, Egerod, Tønnesen, and Lomborg (2012) Study

1. a. Significance of the problem: "Critical illness and admission to the intensive care unit (ICU) radically affects patients and their close relatives during hospitalization and after discharge. Internationally, the long-term consequences of critical illness and ICU admission have been identified as an important professional issue" (Ågård et al., 2012, p. 105).
   b. Background of the problem: "After critical illness, ICU survivors often suffer from disease-specific sequelae, general physical and psychosocial problems requiring considerable efforts to regain pre-ICU functional level (NHS, National Institute for Health and Clinical Excellence, 2009;...). Further, a substantial portion of ICU survivors experience cognitive impairment affecting memory, attention, and executive function (Desai et al., 2011)" (Ågård et al., 2012, p. 106).
   c. Problem statement: "Little is known, however, about the everyday concerns of ICU survivors and their cohabiting partners and the coping modalities employed to meet the challenges facing the couples" (Ågård et al., 2012, p. 106).
2. "The aim [purpose] of the study was to explore the challenges facing ICU survivors with cohabiting spouse or partner and explain patients' concerns

and coping modalities during the first 12 months post ICU discharge" (Ågård et al., 2012, p. 106).

3. The problem is significant since it is recognized as an international professional issue that affects millions of patients and their families. Understanding ICU survivors and their spouses' or partners' experiences postdischarge is a relatively new area of research that is important for nurses to manage. The purpose builds upon the problem statement and clearly indicates the focus of the study.
4. The study purpose clearly identified the research concepts, populations, and settings.
   a. The research concepts are challenges facing ICU survivors and cohabiting spouse or partner and patients' concerns and coping modalities postdischarge ICU.
   b. The populations are ICU survivors and their cohabiting spouse or partner.
   c. The participants were identified in ICUs and probably followed in their homes for 12 months postdischarge.
5. The study was feasible because the researchers have educational, clinical, and research expertise to conduct this study, as was discussed in Chapter 2 of this study guide. The study had several sources of funding indicating strong professional support for the research. The ICUs from three university hospitals and one regional hospital were used to obtain participants, indicating a large pool of potential study participants. The study seemed ethical with potential benefits and limited risks and it had institutional approval and participants provided informed consent.

Objectives, Questions, and Hypotheses

Bindler et al. (2013) Study

1. Bindler et al. (2013, p. 21) stated specific aims or objectives for their study that included: "1. Contrast prevalence of IR and other cardiometabolic risk factors in male and female adolescents; 2. Contrast prevalence of IR and other cardiometabolic risk factors in adolescents according to weight status; 3. Examine correlates of IR with anthropometric and laboratory markers among adolescents; and 4. Determine if lipids/triglycerides, inflammatory markers, and weight status can reliably predict IR in adolescents."
2. The research aims or objectives are clearly stated and direct the development of the design, the data analysis, and interpretation of the findings. This is a correlational study with a comparative descriptive, predictive correlational design. The first research aim focuses on comparative description of prevalence of IR in male and female adolescents. The second aim focuses on comparative description of IR in adolescents based on weight status. Aim 3 focuses on determining relationships between IR and anthropometric and laboratory markers. Aim 4 focuses on identifying variables to predict IR in adolescents.

Knapp et al. (2013) Study

1. This study identified the following objectives: "The objectives were to evaluate the EPICS Family Bundle, change unit culture to one more conducive to family care, and to provide improved care for family members" (Knapp et al., 2013, p. 52).
2. a. These objectives seem more like the goals to be accomplished by a clinical agency than objectives to direct a study. In addition, hypothesis is best developed to direct the conduct of this quasi-experimental study.
   b. The hypothesis might be stated as follows: *Family members provided care by nurses with knowledge of the EPICS Family Bundle have less stress and stronger coping abilities than those family members provided standard nursing care.*

Ågård et al. (2012) Study

1. This is a qualitative study that has no objectives, questions, or hypotheses. The research purpose provides direction for this study, and this is fairly common in qualitative studies.
2. No objectives, questions, or hypotheses

Study Variables or Concepts

Bindler et al. (2013) Study

1. Study variables are identified in Table 3 in the study.

Variable	Type of variable
Age (months)	Independent variable
BMI	Independent variable
BMI percentile	Independent variable
Waist circumference	Independent variable
C-reactive protein (hsCRP)	Independent variable
Triglycerides	Independent variable
Total cholesterol	Independent variable
LDL-C	Independent variable
HDL-C	Independent variable
Systolic blood pressure (SBP)	Independent variable
Diastolic blood pressure (DBP)	Independent variable
Homeostasis Model Assessment of Insulin Resistance (HOMA-IR)	Dependent variable

2. a. Conceptional Definition of HOMA-IR: IR is based on the Homeostasis Model Assessment and is an "indicator of metabolic syndrome (MS) in youth that is related to both longitudinal changes and adiposity" (Bindler et al. 2013, p. 21).
   b. Operational Definition of HOMA-IR: "HOMA-IR was a laboratory calculated value of: insulin (μU/ml) × glucose (mg/dl)/405.0. Lower HOMA-IR scores indicate greater insulin sensitivity, whereas higher HOMA-IR scores reflect greater IR at the cellular level" (Bindler et al. 2013, p. 21).
3. The conceptual and operational definitions for HOMA-IR values are clearly expressed in the study. The conceptual definition provides a strong link to the operational definition, which is exceptionally strong and appropriate for this study. However, the study lacks a clearly identified framework so the conceptual definition lacks a theoretical basis. Adding a physiological/pathological framework would clarify the contribution of these study findings to nursing knowledge.
4. The sample characteristics for this study are presented by gender (male and female) in Table 1 of this research article. The study variables included in the description of the sample were: gender, age, BMI. BMI percentile, waist circumference (cm), HOMA-IR, hsCRP, triglycerides, total cholesterol, LDL-C, HDL-C, SBP, and DBP.

Knapp et al. (2013) Study

1. Study variables

Variable	Type of variable
EPICS Family Bundle educational program provided to the nurses	Independent variable
Stress	Dependent variable
Coping	Dependent variable

2. a. *Conceptual Definition of Stress*: "Lazarus and Folkman view stress as a psychological reaction response and define it as a relationship between a person and the environment that is considered taxing by the person and endangers well-being" (Knapp et al., p. 52).
   b. *Operational Definition of Stress*: Stress was measured with the State-Trait Anxiety Inventory (STAI).
   c. *Conceptual Definition of Coping*: Lazarus and Folkman indicated that "coping consists of cognitive and behavioral efforts to manage stressors" (Knapp et al., p. 52).
   d. *Operational Definition of Coping*: Coping was measured with the Ways of Coping Questionnaire (WAYS).
3. The researchers provided very clear and appropriate conceptual and operational definitions for stress and coping. The conceptual definitions are clearly linked to the study framework, Lazarus and Folkman's Transactional Model of Stress and Coping. The scales used to measure stress and coping are clearly identified and linked to the conceptual definitions. These scales have been used in many studies and have strong reliability and validity.
4. The demographic variables included in this study were: relationship to patient, gender, ethnicity, race, participant (family member) age, patient age, and patient days in the SICU (see Table 1 in the research article).

CHAPTER 6—UNDERSTANDING AND CRITICALLY APPRAISING THE LITERATURE REVIEW

EXERCISE 1: TERMS AND DEFINITIONS

1. m
2. d
3. l
4. n
5. h
6. i
7. c
8. a
9. k
10. j
11. b
12. o
13. f
14. e
15. g

EXERCISE 2: LINKING IDEAS

Examples of Main Ideas from the Chapter

1. (1) relevant; (2) critically appraising; (3) synthesizing
2. known, not known
3. CINAHL
4. 5
5. quantitative
6. ethnographic
7. purpose
8. encyclopedia
9. valid, appropriate
10. regular, italicized

Theoretical and Empirical Sources

1. T
2. E
3. E
4. T
5. T
6. E
7. E
8. E
9. T
10. E

Primary and Secondary Sources

1. S
2. P
3. P
4. P
5. P
6. P
7. S
8. S
9. P
10. P

EXERCISE 3: WEB-BASED INFORMATION AND RESOURCES

1. "White's theory of spirituality and spiritual self-care" (p. 23)
   White, M. (2013). Spiritual self-care effects on quality of life for patients diagnosed with chronic illness. *Self Care & Dependent Care Nursing: The Official Journal of the Orem International Society, 20*(1), 23-32. Retrieved January 17, 2014, from http://www.orem-society.com/images/publication/journal/Vol20No01Spring13.pdf.
2. a. cross-sectional descriptive design
   b. 66.5 months

EXERCISE 4: CONDUCTING CRITICAL APPRAISALS TO BUILD AN EVIDENCE-BASED PRACTICE

1. a. journal title
   b. year of publication
   c. volume number
   d. page numbers
   e. issue number
   f. Sandra J. Knapp
   g. The EPICS Family Bundle and its effects on stress and coping of families of critically ill trauma patients.
2. Bindler, R., Bindler, R., & Daratha, K. (2013). Biological correlates and predictors of insulin resistance among early adolescents. *Journal of Pediatric Nursing, 28*(1), 20-27.
3. a. 2039-2044 (page numbers)
   b. *Hypertension* (journal title)
   c. Fasting and nonfasting lipid levels (article title)
4. a. Review of Literature, Purpose, and Study Aims
   b. Introduction
5. a. Introduction
   b. Discussion
6. Glaser (1978) and Glaser and Strauss (1967)
7. a. Studies were cited, but no theories were cited in the review. The omission of theoretical sources in the review is consistent with grounded theory methodology.
   b. Systematic reviews, books, position statements, clinical articles

8. a. $35/42 = 0.83 \times 100 = 83\%$; $27/42 = 0.64 \times 100 = 64\%$
   b. Cullberg (1993) appears to be a landmark study because it linked intensive care stress and coping to the theories and evidence related to stress and coping in general.
9. a. Medicine, title includes the term "medical task force"
   b. *British Medical Journal* (BMJ)
   c. Yes, although the majority of the citations are from nursing, some are from psychiatry, anesthesiology, and other medical specialties, which indicates that the authors searched medical and health professional databases, in addition to CINAHL.
10. a. Ågård et al. (2012) did not comment on the strength and weaknesses of the studies.
   b. Paragraph 4 of the Introduction: "In summary, recovery can be a strenuous time for both ICU survivors and their close relatives. Little is known, however, about the everyday concerns of ICU survivors and their cohabiting partners and the coping modalities employed to meet the challenges facing the couples. Better insight into these sparsely researched areas could provide healthcare staff with a stronger basis for preparing ICU survivors and their close relatives for post-ICU recovery" (p. 106).
   c. Yes, the review did provide a logical argument for the statement of the research problem. The first premise of the argument is that admission to critical care has a radical effect on patients and families, therefore, the topic is an important professional issue. ICU survivors suffer from long-term health consequences that affect quality of life. Families are affected by the long-term disruption to their lives. Although the argument was clear, the review was not long enough to demonstrate the development of the evidence over time. The researchers did not have space in the article to provide the historical studies that led to those that were cited.
   d. Yes, the main ideas of the literature review were critical illness, CCU admission, stress, challenges, and the consequences of the CCU stay. The purpose includes the same concepts of challenges, concerns, and coping modalities over 12 months. Therefore, the literature summary provided direction for the study purpose.
11. Knapp et al. (2013) described the research related to families of critical care patients, using primarily research reports. They also cited five theory sources with the predominant one being Lazarus and Folkman (1984), a classic theory of stress. Two institutional documents (Marker, 2008; Ziglar, 2008), and three clinical articles (Carter & Clark, 2002; Farvis, 2005; Leon & Knapp, 2002) were cited. Many of the references were 5 to 10 years old (47.6%). A third of the references were over 10 years old; however, included in the older articles were the theoretical sources and others supporting the anxiety instrument. The research report by Molter (1979) appears to be a seminal article. The journals cited were primarily nursing journals, with one being a social work journal and another being a medical journal. Although few references from other disciplines were included, a search of health professional journals revealed that nursing has had a greater interest in family needs than other disciplines. The studies were synthesized, but not critically appraised. The researchers analyzed the studies enough to know and communicate that the intervention studies had not been focused on the effects of nursing education on family needs. There was not summary of the review; rather, in the short introduction, the researchers built an argument to justify the need for the study. The review was not organized chronologically to show the progression of knowledge. Because the researchers included older references for older studies, the reader at least knew that the topic had been of an interest of nurses for many years. Despite using older literature, the literature review provided adequate background to logically support the purpose of the study.

CHAPTER 7—UNDERSTANDING THEORY AND RESEARCH FRAMEWORKS

EXERCISE 1: TERMS AND DEFINITIONS

1. e
2. h
3. a
4. g
5. b
6. f
7. j
8. c
9. i
10. d

EXERCISE 2: LINKING IDEAS

Key Theoretical Ideas

1. variable
2. relational statements
3. hypotheses
4. building blocks

5. Conceptual definitions are abstract, comprehensive definitions based on theory. Operational definitions are narrower and indicate how the variable will be measured, implemented, or observed in the specific study.
6. Grand nursing theories are abstract conceptual models that describe nursing. Middle-range theories are less abstract and focus on a specific phenomenon or situation in practice.
7. practice or prescriptive
8. implicit framework
9. relational statements
10. caring

Levels of Abstraction

Construct (*highest*)
Concept
Variable
Operational definition (*lowest*)

Elements of Theory

1. physical health, psychological health, quality of life
2. relationships between the concepts
3. framework

Examples of Frameworks

1. a
2. c
3. b
4. f
5. h
6. g
7. e
8. d

EXERCISE 3: WEB-BASED INFORMATION AND RESOURCES

1. a. relief, ease, and transcendence
   b. http://currentnursing.com/nursing_theory/comfort_theory_Kathy_Kolcaba.html (URL may vary)
2. a. human capital
   b. relational capital
   c. intellectual capital
   d. structural capital

EXERCISE 4: CONDUCTING CRITICAL APPRAISALS TO BUILD AN EVIDENCE-BASED PRACTICE

Knapp, Sole, and Byers (2013)

1. a. Transactional Cognitive Theory of Stress
   b. Lazarus and Folkman
2. Secondary appraisal

Dickson, Howe, Deal, and McCarthy (2011)

1.

Construct	Concept	Variable(s)
Person	Individual-level factors	1. Depression 2. Physical functioning
Problem	Job-level factors	1. Job demands 2. Job control 3. Workplace support
Environmental	Work Organization	Variables for this concept were not clearly separated from the variables for job-level factors
Behavior (implied construct)	Self-care	1. Adherence to recommended behaviors
Outcome (implied construct)	Quality of life	1. Health-related quality of life 2. General quality of life

2. Situation-specific theory of heart failure self-care
3. Orem's theory of self-care

Allen, Ploeg, and Kaasalainen (2012)

1. ***Emotional intelligence*** is "non-cognitive capabilities, competencies, and skill" (p. 231) or a "mixture of emotion-related competencies, personality traits, and character…" (p. 232), affecting coping, adaptability, and succeeding in interaction with self and others (defined in slightly different ways in different parts of the article).
   Clinical teaching effectiveness, as defined by Knox and Morgan (1985), is the actions and learning activities initiated by the teacher to enhance students' learning in a clinical environment.
2. a. Model of Social-Emotional Intelligence
   b. Bar-On (2005)
3.

Emotional intelligence	Clinical teaching effectiveness
a. Intrapersonal b. Interpersonal c. Stress management d. Adaptability e. General mood	a. Teaching ability b. Nursing competence c. Evaluation d. Interpersonal relationships e. Personality trait

Bindler, Bindler, and Daratha (2013)

1. Scientific theory
2. Answers may vary. The answers below are provided as examples.

Variable	Conceptual definition	Operational definition
Obesity	Body weight greater than established standard	Computation of BMI
Serum lipids	Fat-like components in blood that influence the formation of plaque in blood vessels	Quantification of cholesterol and triglycerides based on the analysis of fasting blood sample

Piamjariyakul, Smith, Russell, Werkowitch, and Elyachar (2013)

1. Relationships between coaching strategies and intermediate outcomes that have been empirically verified in published studies
2. It means that the process of coaching by professionals is supported by evidence-based clinical guidelines.
3. a. Confidence in providing heart failure care (intermediate outcome)
   b. Preparedness (intermediate outcome)
   c. Caregiver burden (long-term outcome)

CHAPTER 8—CLARIFYING QUANTITATIVE RESEARCH DESIGNS

EXERCISE 1: TERMS AND DEFINITIONS

Understanding Common Design Terms

1. a
2. m
3. b
4. e
5. d
6. c
7. j
8. i
9. f
10. g
11. k
12. h
13. n
14. l

Design Validity Terms

1. b
2. e
3. a
4. f
5. h
6. i
7. c
8. j
9. d
10. g

EXERCISE 2: LINKING IDEAS

1. effects or outcomes
2. cause; effect or outcome; cause
3. treatment, intervention, or independent variable
4. cause and effect, causality, or the effect of a treatment on a study outcome
5. control
6. experimental design
7. design validity
8. multicausality and also a predictive correlational design
9. intervention or treatment
10. intervention fidelity
11. control
12. descriptive and correlational studies, also called nonexperimental studies
13. comparative descriptive
14. Correlational
15. model testing
16. You might include any of the following:
    a. an experimental or treatment group receives the study treatment or intervention
    b. usually includes a control or comparison group
    c. control of the setting
    d. manipulation of an independent variable or intervention by the researchers
    e. control of extraneous variables
    f. random assignment of subjects to groups
    g. random selection of subjects if possible
17. large samples

Determining Types of Design Validity in Studies

1. d
2. a
3. b
4. d
5. c
6. b
7. c
8. d
9. c
10. a

Identifying a Design Model

1. A model of a typical descriptive design with four study variables is presented in Chapter 8 in Figure 8-3 of your textbook, *Understanding Nursing Research*, 6th edition.
2. A descriptive correlational design model is presented in Figure 8-6 of your textbook.
3. Quasi-experimental pretest and posttest design with comparison group model is presented in Figure 8-9 of your textbook.

Control and Designs for Nursing Studies

1. Quasi-experimental posttest-only design with comparison group—used to examine the effect of an animated program provided on DVD to ensure the fidelity of the intervention. The study included

only a posttest to measure pain with the FACES scale following the DVD viewing and IV insertion. The FACES scale is a quality method for measuring pain in children. The age of the children was controlled, as was the setting for the study. The children were obtained by a sample of convenience and were not randomly assigned to groups, but the groups were equal in number. There is possible threat to internal design validity since the children were placed in a group based on their hospital unit and these units might be different in some way.

2. Randomized controlled trial (RCT)—testing the effectiveness of a new hypertensive medication. The study has a large sample size with random assignment to the comparison and experimental groups. The study was conducted in multiple sites and two different geographical areas. In addition, the medication intervention was manipulated in a controlled way to ensure the right subject got the medication and that the medication was delivered accurately at the right time, right dose, and right route. Measurement of BP was controlled to ensure precise and accurate readings.
3. Correlational study—The relationships among the variables of hours of sleep, stress level, anxiety level, and depression were measured in first-time mothers. The sample was limited to first-time mothers in the first month following the birth of their child. Often correlational studies have limited controls so the population might be studied without manipulation in a natural setting.
4. Descriptive study—The study focused on identifying the health promotion and illness prevention behaviors of patients experiencing their first myocardial infarction (MI). The only control is the limitation of sample to patients with their first MI. Most descriptive studies include limited control to ensure the study variables are described as they occur naturally in the world.
5. Comparative descriptive design—describing and examining the differences between males' and females' health promotion behaviors. The study population is people with diabetes who were studied in clinics with no manipulation of the setting.
6. Quasi-experimental pretest and posttest design with comparison group—examining the effects of vitamins on infant weight gain. The pretest was done prior to implementing the vitamin intervention, and the posttest was conducted at 6 months of age. The intervention of vitamins was controlled by using a detailed protocol for implementation. The sample was one of convenience obtained from three pediatricians' offices, and the subjects were randomly assigned to the intervention and comparison groups.
7. Model testing design—testing the use of the Orem Self-Care Model to predict self-care behaviors in diabetic adolescents. The study was limited to adolescents, but no other controls were evident in the study.
8. Predictive correlational design—the study examines measurement of perception of self-esteem, depression level, age, and educational level to predict the self-care abilities of women being treated for lung cancer. This correlation study identified a specific population, but the study was conducted with minimal controls to examine the relationships as they naturally exist in the world.

EXERCISE 3: WEB-BASED INFORMATION AND RESOURCES

1. a. Farrell and Shafiei (2012) indicated that they used a descriptive design in conducting their study.
   b. Data were collected using questionnaires that were mailed to nurses identified through the Nurses Board of Victoria.
2. a. "Quasi-experimental, one-group, pretest–posttest design" was identified in the study (Aronson et al., 2013, p. e124).
   b. Yes, the study included the Role-Modeling Intervention. "The Role-Modeling Intervention consists of a 40-minute expert practice video, combined with verbal reinforcement of expected behaviors and tailored feedback" (Aronson et al., 2013, p. e123).
   c. The data collection process was highly structured and detailed in the study in Figure 1 and in the Procedures section (see p. e124).

EXERCISE 4: CONDUCTING CRITICAL APPRAISALS TO BUILD AN EVIDENCE-BASED PRACTICE

Bindler, Bindler, and Daratha (2013)

Answers address the critical appraisal for the design of the Bindler et al. (2013) study in Appendix B.

1. The Bindler et al. (2013) study has a predictive correlational design. The purpose identifies the type of design: The purposes in the "Mentoring in School (TEAMS) study were to describe the anthropometric and laboratory markers of participants and to test the ability of these markers to **predict** risk of exhibiting IR [insulin resistance]" (Bindler et al., 2013, p. 21). The study aims or objectives also supported this design. See Chapter 5 for a discussion of these objectives.

2. Insulin resistance (IR) is the *dependent* variable predicted in this study.
3. The independent variables of anthropometric markers (BMI, BMI percentile, and waist circumference); laboratory markers (total cholesterol, low density lipoprotein-cholesterol [LDL-C], high-density lipoprotein-cholesterol [HDL-C], triglycerides, and C-reactive protein [hsCRP]); and systolic and diastolic blood pressures (BPs) were used to predict the dependent variable IR in this study.
4. Bindler et al.'s (2013) study mainly focused on relationships, but the researchers did make comparisons between the males and females for all study variables (see Table 1). The subjects were also divided into two groups based on BMI percentiles, those <95th BMI percentile and those ≥95th BMI percentile, and differences in the variables were examined for these two groups (see Table 2).
5. You might have identified any of the following design validity strengths from this study.
   a. "Fasting serum venipunctures were performed by licensed phlebotomists in early morning" (Bindler et al., 2013, p. 21), ensuring these data were consistently collected by trained professionals to promote precision and accuracy of the laboratory values. The study has strong construct design validity, with the variables measured in the study being clearly conceptually and operationally defined.
   b. Anthropometric measurements were obtained by trained personnel to promote precise and accurate measurements of BMI and waist circumference. The details for measurements are provided in the article.
   c. The BMI was examined as a single value and a percentile strengthening the construct validity of the study. Three cholesterol values (total, LDL-C, and HDL-C) were measured based on laboratory standards, avoiding mono-operational bias.
   d. The BPs were measured using protocols from the National Health and Nutrition Examination Survey, ensuring consistent measurement based on a national standard. The details for BP measurements are also listed in the study, construct design validity strength.
   e. The sample size was strong with 150 participants, decreasing the potential for low statistical power.
   f. The data were collected at one point in time (baseline), and there was no subject attrition or history or maturation effects, which strengthen the internal design validity of the study.
6. Threats to design validity: You might have identified any of the following ideas, or you might have identified other threats in the Bindler et al. (2013) study.
   a. The predictive correlational design used in the study was not clearly identified and had to be determined based on the purpose and the study aims.
   b. The sample was not randomly selected; it was a nonprobability sample of convenience. Nonrandom sample decreases the potential to generalize the findings.
   c. The groups were of unequal size when examining differences based on gender and BMI percentile. Only 39 adolescents were in the ≥95th BMI percentile and 111 were in the <95th BMI percentile. The small numbers in the ≥95th percentile group might have affected the results, and limits the understanding for this group of adolescents. The number of males was 64 and the number of females was 86, which might have also affected the study results.
   d. IR was measured with only one method, resulting in mono-operational bias; however, the measurement was the national standard, making this a minimal weakness.
   e. No power analysis was addressed to determine the sample size needed for the study. Was the sample size large enough to prevent a Type II error?
7. You may have identified any of the following methods of control in the Bindler et al. (2013) study.
   a. Controlling measurement of all physiological variables including anthropometric and laboratory markers, BP, and IR.
   b. Controlling extraneous variables: Blood draws were done in early morning by a licensed phlebotomist after the subjects had fasted.
   c. Controlling environment: All measurements were completed in 1 day at the same setting.
   d. Controlling mono-operational bias: Used multiple measures for most of the variables.
   e. Controlling for the effects of maturation: Fed students after fasting blood draws so that increasing hunger did not affect study results.
   f. Control of the ethical aspects of the study such as institutional review board approval and obtaining informed consent from the subjects.
8. Generalization is limited to adolescents who are similar to the students taking part in the TEAMS study. Also, the number of adolescents with ≥95th BMI percentile have limited representation, which decreases the generalization of the findings to these individuals. Additional research is needed to determine the independent variables predictive of IR in adolescents.

Knapp, Sole, and Byers (2013)

Answers address the critical appraisal of the design of the Knapp, Sole, and Byers (2013) study found in Appendix C.

1. Type of design: "A quasi-experimental design, nonequivalent control group, pretest-posttest design was used to conduct this study" (Knapp et al., 2013, p. 52).
2. The intervention implemented in this study was the EPICS Family Bundle that was developed to improve the interactions of nurses with family members of critically Ill trauma patients.
3. Comparisons made in the Knapp et al. (2013) study are described as follows: Because this was a quasi-experimental study focused on determining the effects of a treatment on selected dependent variables and included only one group, the comparisons were between the pretest and posttest measurements. The pretest was conducted on 39 family members (identified as the control group) and the posttest was conducted using 45 family members (identified as the experimental group). It is unclear whether some of these were the same family members in the pretest and posttest, since data were collected over 3 months. The dependent variables compared were stress and coping, which were measured prior to and after the intervention.
4. Strengths in the Knapp et al. (2013) study design include the following:
   a. EPICS Family Bundle Intervention had strong, relevant content. "The program was designed as a computer-based course that met state requirements for trauma-related continuing education (two contact hours)" (Knapp et al., 2013, p. 53).
   b. EPICS intervention was pilot-tested to ensure consistency in its implementation, statistical conclusion validity strength.
   c. The researchers and other key staff nurses who worked in the SICU championed the intervention and encouraged nurses to participate to increase the number of nurses exposed to the EPICS intervention.
   d. Anxiety had a clear conceptual definition based on the study framework and a strong operational definition (construct design validity strength). Anxiety was measured with the State Trait Anxiety Inventory (STAI) that was developed in 1983 and has been used in many studies. The scale was reliable in previous studies and also in this study (statistical conclusion design validity strength).
   e. Coping had a clear conceptual definition based on the study framework and a strong operational definition (construct validity strength). Coping was measured with the Ways of Coping Questionnaire (WAYS) that was developed in 1988 and has been reliable when used in previous studies (statistical conclusion validity strength).
   f. The demographic variables for the pretest (control) and posttest (experimental) groups were examined for differences, and no significant differences were found (see Table 1), decreasing the potential effects from extraneous variables.
   g. One controlled setting, a 30-bed SICU, was used for the study, decreasing the potential for an interaction between the setting and treatment and the effect of extraneous variables (external validity strength).
5. Threats to design validity for the Knapp et al. (2013) study include the following:
   a. The nonequivalent pretest-posttest control group design is a weak design. The study would have been stronger if it included both an experimental group and comparison group.
   b. The sample included 84 family members, but the power analysis indicated that a sample size of 134 was needed with 67 in each group. The pretest group had only 39 subjects and the posttest group had 45 subjects. Therefore, this study had low statistical power, and the nonsignificant findings for stress and coping might have been due to a Type II error (threat to statistical conclusion validity).
   c. There was no random assignment of subjects to groups, resulting in possible threat to internal design validity.
   d. The original sample was not random, and there is a potential for sampling bias with a nonprobability sample of convenience.
   e. Both anxiety and coping were measured with only one scale, resulting in mono-operational bias.
   f. The specific reliability for the WAYS scale was not presented in this study. The researchers only indicated that the scale reliability was comparable to previous studies.
   g. The validity information for both the STAI and WAYS scales was limited in the study and a potential threat to construct design validity.
   h. Only 52 (43%) of the 120 nurses in the SICU completed the EPICS intervention that was designated by management as optional, which is a strong threat to the design validity of this study. Several nurses did not support the use of this intervention in the SICU and did not do the training. It is unclear how the study was managed to ensure that the families included

in the study interacted with the nurses who had been trained with the intervention.

6. Methods of control used in the Knapp et al. (2013) study design that you might have identified include the following:
   a. Extensive control of the EPICS intervention content and implementation. Intervention was pilot-tested to identify potential problems. However, the lack of nurses' participation in the intervention reduced the effect of the intervention.
   b. Details on the methods used to obtain nurses' participation in the study.
   c. Control of the measurement of anxiety and coping.
   d. Control of the ethical aspects of the study such as institutional review board approval and obtaining informed consent from the subjects.
7. The researchers did not generalize the study findings. They recognized the limitations of the study, such as the small sample size, nonsignificant findings, and the fact that only 52 (43%) of 120 of the staff members in the SICU completed the EPICS intervention. Additional research is needed to determine the effectiveness of the EPICS intervention.

CHAPTER 9—EXAMINING POPULATIONS AND SAMPLES IN RESEARCH

EXERCISE 1: TERMS AND DEFINITIONS

1. j
2. a
3. n
4. g
5. k
6. f
7. m
8. i
9. l
10. b
11. d
12. e
13. h
14. c
15. o

EXERCISE 2: LINKING IDEAS

1. elements
2. target population
3. sample, accessible population, and target population
4. You might identify any of the following:
   a. Compare the demographic characteristics of the sample with those of the target population determined from previous research.
   b. Compare mean sample values of study variables with the values of the target population determined from previous research.
   c. Identify the refusal rate in the study and identify the reasons potential subjects refused to participate. The lower the refusal rate and the more common the reasons for refusing to participate, the more representative the sample is of the target population.
   d. Evaluate the possibilities of systematic bias in the sample in terms of the setting, characteristics of the sample, and ranges of values on measured variables.
   e. Determine sample attrition rate and identify the reasons for the attrition or withdrawal of subjects from the study. The lower the attrition rate and the more common or usual the reasons for attrition, the more representative the sample is of the target population.
5. the expected difference in values that occurs when different subjects from the same sample are examined
6. sampling frame
7. strategies or method(s) used to obtain a sample for a study
8. You might choose any of the following:
   a. Was the sampling plan adequately identified?
   b. Did the researcher successfully implement the sampling plan?
   c. Was the sampling plan effective in achieving representativeness of the target population?
   d. Were the subjects or participants selected from a sampling frame?
   e. Were the subjects or participants randomly selected?
9. homogeneous
10. heterogeneous
11. sampling criteria
12. sample characteristics
13. sample attrition
14. a. simple random sampling
    b. stratified random sampling
    c. cluster sampling
    d. systematic sampling
15. You might list any of the following:
    a. convenience sampling
    b. network sampling
    c. purposive sampling
    d. theoretical sampling
16. nonprobability
17. power analysis
18. differences or relationships
19. 0.8 or 80%
20. null hypothesis

21. You might list any of the following:
    a. effect size of a study
    b. type of study
    c. number of variables
    d. measurement sensitivity
    e. data analysis techniques
22. You might list any of the following:
    a. data saturation
    b. scope of the study
    c. nature of the topic
    d. quality of the information
    e. study design
23. inclusion and exclusion
24. Refusal number = 250 – 208 = 42. Refusal rate = 42 refused ÷ 250 subjects approached = 0.168 × 100% = 16.8%
25. Attrition rate = 20 withdrew from the study ÷ 150 sample size = 0.133 × 100% = 13.3%

Sampling Methods for Quantitative and Qualitative Studies

1. f	11. f
2. b	12. c
3. c	13. d
4. a	14. b
5. b	15. f
6. g	16. h
7. h	17. i
8. b	18. a
9. e	19. d
10. d	20. b

Determining Sample Size for Quantitative and Qualitative Studies

1. a	6. b
2. c	7. c
3. b	8. b
4. a	9. a
5. b	10. b

EXERCISE 3: WEB-BASED INFORMATION AND RESOURCES

1. The Aronson et al. (2013) study can be located on the Elsevier website for the textbook, http://evolve.elsevier.com/grove/understanding/. Find this article and review the sampling section. Also review the other information that is provided on this website.
    a. convenience sample
    b. Sample size was $N = 24$, or 12 student dyads
2. The Coker-Bolt et al. (2013) study can be located on the Elsevier website for the textbook, http://evolve.elsevier.com/grove/understanding/.
    a. The specific sampling method is not identified in the study. However, it appears that the researchers used a sample of convenience since the infants were identified from the Medical University of South Carolina (MUSC) Division of Pediatric Cardiology patient database. It is important that researchers identify their sampling method in their research report.
    b. The sample size for this study was 28 (see narrative p. 66 and Table 1).
    c. Treatment group had 18 infants ($n = 18$) and the comparison group has 10 infants ($n = 10$) (see narrative p. 66 and Table 1).
    d. The sample sizes for the treatment and comparison groups were small and very unequal, which could lead to errors in the study results. The researchers found a significant difference between the groups for length of stay (LOS), but not between the groups on the time to achieve full bottle-feeds. The sample size was large enough for LOS; however, the effect sizes for the other variables were probably smaller and the sample size was not adequate to assure that a Type II error did not occur. The study would have been strengthened by a larger sample with random and equal assignment of infants to either the treatment group or comparison group. A larger sample would reduce the potential for a Type II error of saying something is not significant when it is.
3. You might have identified a variety of websites that discussed power analysis. For example, the following website posted at UCLA (University of California at Los Angeles) provides a discussion of power analysis: http://www.ats.ucla.edu/stat/seminars/Intro_power/.

    G*Power provides an online program for understanding and conducting power analysis. Locate the free software at http://www.softpedia.com/get/Science-CAD/G-Power.shtml.

    Some websites have useful information about research methodology; however, review the websites for quality of information. University websites usually provide more credible information than websites advertising products or services. Some websites will direct you to research articles and books that focus on power analysis and these could be excellent sources of information.

EXERCISE 4: CONDUCTING CRITICAL APPRAISALS TO BUILD AN EVIDENCE-BASED PRACTICE

Bindler, Bindler, and Daratha (2013) Study

1. Population was early adolescents or might have identified middle school students.
2. Inclusion sample criteria were: "Participants included all middle school students who volunteered to participate in a project called TEAMS" (p. 21). Exclusion sample criteria: "Students with mental or physical conditions that would limit their participation in study activities or those taking insulin or oral glycemic medications were excluded" (p. 21).
3. The sample characteristics for the participants were presented in Table 1, Sample Characteristics by Gender (p. 22), and Table 2, Sample Characteristics by Weight Status (p. 23).
4. Sample size was 150 adolescents ($N = 150$) with $n = 64$ males and $n = 86$ females (see Table 1).
5. The sample size was fairly large at 150 adolescents. However, the study did include examination of several variables and the sorting of participants into gender and BMI groups for analysis, which require increased study participants. No power analysis was conducted to determine an adequate sample size for this type of study and the number of variables and groups examined. The lack of a power analysis to determine the sample size limits the ability of the reader to judge the adequacy of the sample size.
6. There is no indication of sample attrition since the original sample size was 150 adolescents and all data analyses were conducted on 150 participants. Having no attrition of study participants is a study strength.
7. Nonprobability sampling
8. The sampling method is not identified in the article, but appears to be a sample of convenience since all middle school students participating in a TEAMS Project were included in the study.
9. The representativeness of the sample is limited because only the students participating in the TEAMS Project were included in the study and they might be different in some way from those not participating in the project. In addition, a nonrandom sampling method was used to obtain the sample. The sample was 57% female so was more representative of females than males in the population. However, the study seems to have 0% refusal and attrition rates, which increase the representativeness of the sample.
10. The generalization of the study findings is decreased by the nonprobability sampling method and the limited representativeness of the sample. However, because some of these study findings were consistent with the findings of other studies, this increases the generalizability of the findings. Because this is a relatively new area of research for adolescents, the findings can be generalized to the sample and probably the accessible population, but not to the target population. Additional research is needed in this problem area before the findings are ready for generalization to the target population.
11. The settings for this study were the adolescent students' "respective schools or at the university campus" (p. 21). These seem to be natural settings for the students to facilitate data collection.

Knapp, Sole, and Byers (2013) Study

1. The population is family members of critically ill trauma patients.
2. Sampling inclusion criteria: "Participants were family members of critically ill trauma patients who had been admitted to the surgical intensive care unit (SICU) for at least 48 hours. Family members were at least 18 years old; spouse, parent, child, sibling, or significant other; and able to read and complete study tools in English" (p. 53). No sample exclusion criteria were identified.
3. "Sample characteristics: Data were collected on 39 family members in the control group and 45 in the intervention group. Average age for participants and patients ranged from 46 to 50; and the duration of patient hospitalization at the time of the study was 4.5 days. Demographic data for the sample are shown in Table 1 (p. 54). No differences ($p > .05$) were noted in characteristics of participants in the control and intervention groups: age, gender, relationship to patient, ethnicity, and race. Likewise, no differences were noted in the patients' characteristics of age and duration of hospitalization in SICU" (p. 54). No difference in the groups' sample characteristics is a study strength, indicating the participants in the two groups were similar at the start of the study and any significant differences found after the intervention is implemented are thought to be caused by the intervention and not chance or error.
4. Sample size was 84 family members with 39 in the control group and 45 in the experimental or intervention group. Sample size was clearly identified in the study abstract (p. 51).
5. Power analysis was conducted to determine the sample size needed for the study. "The target sample size was 134 participants (67 in each group). Sample size estimates were based on an independent sample t-test assuming a medium effect size, alpha = .05, and power .80" (p. 53).
6. No, the sample size was not adequate in this study. The sample size achieved was 84 and the power

analysis indicated that a sample of 134 participants was needed. In addition, only significant differences were noted for distancing and accepting responsibility subsets of coping between the experimental group receiving the EPICS Family Bundle intervention and the control group receiving standard care. There were no significant differences in family stress and for most of the subsets of coping between the intervention and the control group. These nonsignificant results could be due to the inadequate sample size causing a Type II error. The researchers also identified the low sample size as a limitation of the study and provided a rationale for the limited number of study participants.

7. The study identifies a sample size of 84 and analyses were conducted on 84 participants, indicating no attrition of study participants.
8. nonprobability sampling
9. convenience sample
10. The sample is not representative of the target populations studied. The sample size was too small based on the power analysis results, the sampling method was not random, and the group sizes were unequal, which decrease the probability of the sample being representative of the target population. However, a strength of the study is that the groups were similar for demographic characteristics at the start of the study.
11. Since the sample size is small, the sampling method is not random, and many of the findings are not significant, the researchers need to limit the generalization of their findings to the sample. The study needs to be repeated with a larger sample before generalizing to the accessible or target populations.
12. "The study was conducted in the 30-bed SICU at a 617-bed tertiary university medical center in north central Florida with a level-1 trauma center" (p. 53). This hospital is typical of a partially controlled setting.

Ågård, Egerod, Tønnesen, and Lomborg (2012) Study

1. The population was intensive care unit (ICU) survivors.
2. The researchers included detailed sample inclusion and exclusion criteria to decrease the heterogeneity of the ICU-population studied. "To avoid some of the problems of heterogeneity, our inclusion criteria were quite narrow: (1) ICU survivors aged 25-70 years (people of working age), (2) intubation > 96 hours (to target the more severely ill patients)… (3) patients with cohabiting partner (potential primary caregiver after discharge), and (4) ability to communicate adequately in Danish.

   To minimize the impact of prior illness on post-ICU recovery, we excluded patients with conditions that might have severely affected the patients' daily life prior to ICU admission… In addition to patients with major heart, lung, (e.g. chronic obstructive pulmonary disease), or neurological disease, we also excluded patients with conditions such as depression, brain damage, schizophrenia, cancer, a recent history of drug/alcohol abuse prior to admission, or after attempted suicide. Finally, the patient was excluded if a pre-admission health status was missing in the hospital chart" (p. 106).
3. Sample characteristics: "Patient characteristics are provided in Table 1 [p. 108] to illustrate the context of everyday post-ICU recovery. Patients were aged 35-70 years; 11 were men, 7 women. The ICU survivors, who were all generally in good health prior to critical illness, reported a wide range of complications the first year after ICU discharge. The majority had experienced weight loss (5-25 kilos), fatigue, and loss of appetite" (p. 107).
4. Sample included 18 patients and their partners ($n = 18 + 18) = 36$ participants or 18 dyads.
5. The sample size seems adequate for this grounded theory study. The researchers detailed their data collection process using individual and group interviews at 3 months and 12 months post ICU discharge. The researchers noted: "During the 12-month interviews, we coded both selectively and theoretically, while we further tested our ideas and looked for changes in concerns over time, while gradually saturating our substantive grounded theory" (p. 107). The saturation of the theory indicates adequate sample for this study.
6. The researchers noted that they had "18 patients and their partners at three ($n = 18 + 18$) and 12 (n = 17 +16) months post ICU discharge. One couple and one partner withdrew from the study before the 12-month interview" (p. 107). The attrition of the three participants is also noted in Figure 1, titled Patient and Caregiver Enrollment (p. 107). The attrition rate = 3 ÷ 36 = 0.0833 x 100% = 8.33%.
7. Nonprobability sampling method was used in the study.
8. "convenience sample from 5 ICUs" (p. 106).
9. Generalization of findings is not the focus of qualitative research. The focus of grounded theory research is the development of a theory to describe a situation, event, or experience. In this study, the focus was on development of a theory on the convalescence of ICU survivors 12 months post ICU discharge.
10. The study participants were identified over a 10-month period from five ICUs. The individual interviews took place in the couples' home or

in a quiet room at the hospital. The focus group interviews took place at one of the hospitals. These are natural settings that allow the participants a comfortable place to share information.

CHAPTER 10—CLARIFYING MEASUREMENT AND DATA COLLECTION IN QUANTITATIVE RESEARCH

EXERCISE 1: TERMS AND DEFINITIONS

Measurement Concepts and Methods

1. g
2. m
3. i
4. e
5. j
6. h
7. o
8. a
9. d
10. c
11. b
12. n
13. f
14. k
15. l

Reliability, Validity, Accuracy, and Precision in Measurement

1. m
2. a
3. k
4. e
5. g
6. l
7. j
8. d
9. c
10. i
11. f
12. h
13. b

Data Collection

1. d
2. b
3. c
4. e
5. a
6. f

EXERCISE 2: LINKING IDEAS

1. ratio level of measurement
2. 0.8
3. exhaustive and exclusive
4. unequal, equal
5. a self-report form designed to elicit information through written, verbal, or electronic responses from the subject
6. interval
7. 1.00
8. reliable
9. Cronbach's alpha
10. it is not valid
11. reliability and validity
12. unstructured
13. structured
14. personal interview
15. rating
16. visual analog scale
17. You might have listed any of the following or might have another idea that results in measurement error.
    a. Poorly constructed scale or questionnaire that lacks reliability and validity.
    b. Physiological measurement method that lacks precision and accuracy, like inaccurate blood pressure equipment.
    c. Variations in administration of the measurement method.
    d. Subjects leaving an item blank accidentally on a measurement scale.
    e. Hitting the wrong key when entering data into the computer.
    f. Subjects completing a paper-and-pencil scale accidentally marking the wrong column.
    g. Subjects misreading an item on a measurement method.

Measurement Error

1. b
2. b
3. a
4. b
5. a

Levels of Measurement

1. c
2. a
3. b
4. d
5. a
6. b
7. d
8. a
9. b or c
10. d
11. d
12. d
13. b
14. d
15. d
16. d
17. a
18. a
19. b
20. a

Scales

1. a
2. c
3. b

Sensitivity and Specificity

1.

Diagnostic test results	Disease present	Disease not present or absent
Positive test	*a* (true positive)	*b* (false positive)
Negative test	*c* (false negative)	*d* (true negative)

2. Formula for sensitivity: $a/(a + c)$ = True positive rate
3. Formula for specificity: $d/(b + d)$ = True negative rate

Sensitivity and Specificity of Colonoscopy Screening Tests

4. 55
5. 55 ÷ 305 = 0.1803 × 100% = 18.03%
6. 50
7. 50 ÷ 800 = 0.0625 × 100% = 6.25%
8. Sensitivity = 250/(250 + 50) = 250/300 = 0.8333 × 100 = 83.33%
9. Specificity = 750/(55 + 750) = 750/805 = 0.9317 × 100% = 93.17%
10. Positive LR = sensitivity ÷ (100% – specificity)
11. Positive LR = 83.33% ÷ (100% – 93.17%) = 83.33% ÷ 6.83% = 12.20
12. Negative LR = (100% – sensitivity) ÷ specificity
13. Negative LR = (100% – 83.33%) ÷ 93.17% = 16.67% ÷ 93.17% = 0.179 = 0.18

EXERCISE 3: WEB-BASED INFORMATION AND RESOURCES

1. http://www.qualitymeasures.ahrq.gov/
2. You might have identified any of the following websites or others that discuss the CES-D:
   http://cesd-r.com/
   http://counsellingresource.com/lib/quizzes/depression-testing/cesd/
   http://apm.sagepub.com/content/1/3/385.abstract
3. You might have identified one of the following websites:
   http://www.ncbi.nlm.nih.gov/pubmed/2301363
   http://ajp.psychiatryonline.org/article.aspx?articleid=163493
4. http://www.wongbakerfaces.org/
5. You might have identified one of the following websites: http://www.apa.org/pi/about/publications/caregivers/practice-settings/assessment/tools/trait-state.aspx
   http://en.wikipedia.org/wiki/State-Trait_Anxiety_Inventory

   Wikipedia has some good information, but be sure to identify more professional sources to document in your assignments.
6. http://www.mindgarden.com/products/staisad.htm

   The Internet provides extensive information about the instruments used in a variety of nursing studies.

EXERCISE 4: CONDUCTING CRITICAL APPRAISALS TO BUILD AN EVIDENCE-BASED PRACTICE

Bindler, Bindler, and Daratha (2013) Study

1. Bindler et al. (2013) study: Measurement methods and directness of measurement.

Variable(s)	Measurement method(s)	Direct or indirect measurement method
Insulin resistance (IR)	Homeostasis Model Assessments of Insulin Resistance (HOMA-IR)	Indirect measure
Total cholesterol (TC), high-density lipoprotein-cholesterol (HDL-C), and low-density lipoprotein-cholesterol (LDL-C)	Laboratory blood draw	Direct measure
Body mass index (BMI)	"BMI was calculated by dividing weight in pounds by height in inches squared, and multiplying by a conversion factor of 703" (Bindler et al., 2013, p. 21).	Indirect measure
Blood pressure (BP): SBP and DBP	Cuff, stethoscope, and sphygmomanometer	Direct measure

2. Bindler et al. (2013) study: Precision and accuracy of measurement methods.

Variable(s) and measurement methods	Precision and accuracy information from study
HOMA-IR	"HOMA-IR was chosen as the method for measuring IR in this study because it is recognized as a reliable test for IR, is a strong indicator of metabolic syndrome (MS) in youth, and is related to both longitudinal changes and adiposity… HOMA-IR was calculated as insulin (μU/ml) × glucose (mg/dl)/405.0. Lower HOMA-IR scores indicate greater insulin sensitivity, whereas higher HOMA-IR scores indicate greater IR at the cellular level" (precision and accuracy) (Bindler et al., 2013, p. 21).
Blood pressure (BP): Cuff, stethoscope, and sphygmomanometer	SBP and DBP "were measured using the protocols of the National Health and Nutrition Examination Survey (NHANES: CDC, 2005). Research participants sat quietly for 5 minutes. The largest cuff that would fit on the upper arm and leave room below for the head of the stethoscope was chosen, and the participant sat with right arm supported on a table at heart level. The radial pulse was palpated while inflating the cuff, and the level at which the pulse was not palpated was noted; the cuff was then fully deflated. With the stethoscope on the brachial artery, the BP cuff was inflated to 20-30 mm Hg above the level of cessation of the radial pulse. The cuff was deflated 2 mm Hg per second noting the SBP and DBP. For two additional times, the participant sat quietly for 2 minutes, and the BP was measured again. As recommended by NHANES, the first BP measurement was not used in calculation; the remaining two SBP and DBP readings were averaged for use in the study" (Bindler et al., 2013, pp. 21-22).

3. Bindler et al. (2013) provided excellent descriptions of the precision and accuracy of the HOMA-IR and BP measures.
   HOMA-IR calculation was described and rationale was provided for why it was the most precise and accurate measure of IR in youth. The lower and upper scores for HOMA-IR were described.
   SBP and DBP were measured precisely and accurately using a protocol from NHANES. The details for taking BPs were described and three BP readings were taken with the average of the second and third readings used in the study. Multiple readings of participants' BPs using a national standardized protocol increased the precision and accuracy of the BP values obtained for the study.
4. These researchers provided a detailed description of measurement methods and data collection in the section titled "Procedures" in their study. "University and school district institutional review board approvals and signed parent permission/student assent were obtained…
   Fasting serum venipunctures were performed by licensed phlebotomists in early morning, followed by a nutritious breakfast…
   Anthropometric measurement of students by trained personnel included height and weight…
   BP percentiles were reached using the National Heart, Lung, and Blood Institute BP tables, which take into account the height percentile, gender, and age of participants" (Bindler et al., 2013, pp. 21-22).
5. Bindler et al. (2013) indicated IRB approval for the study and that permission was obtained from the parents and assent from the students. They provided excellent detail about the precision and accuracy of the physiological measures used in the study and how data were rigorously collected using protocols based on national standards. The consistency of data collection was promoted with the use of highly qualified professionals who were trained for reliability in the data collection process.

Knapp, Sole, and Byers (2013) Study

1. Knapp et al. (2013) measurement methods and directness of measurement.

Variable(s)	Measurement method(s)	Direct or indirect measurement method
Stress	State-Trait Anxiety Inventory (STAI)	Indirect measure
Coping	Ways of Coping Questionnaire (WAYS)	Indirect measure

2. Knapp et al. (2013) reliability and validity for measurement methods.

Variable(s) and measurement methods	Reliability and validity information from study
Stress: STAI	"The STAI has been used in many studies to measure the effects of an intervention on stress or anxiety in a variety of populations, including families of the critically ill. It is self-reporting tool consisting of 40 statements: 20 related to state anxiety, and 20 related to trait anxiety with higher scores representing higher anxiety. A four point Likert-type rating scale is used… Cronbach's alpha for the normative studies was consistently greater than .86, verifying internal consistency (Spielberger, 1983). In this study, the Cronbach's alpha was .92 for both state and trait anxiety. Test-retest reliability was assessed in the study population by administering the instruments twice on the same day to two participants. Agreement was 98% with both participants" (Knapp et al., 2013, p. 53).
Coping: WAYS	"WAYS is a self-reporting tool that is widely used to assess coping. It consists of 66 items and uses a four-point Likert-type scale. Eight coping subscales are derived from 50 items on the tool. Internal consistency of the WAYS ranges from 0.61 to 0.79. Possible scores range from 0 to 198, with higher scores representing more use of coping skills. The tool is recommended by the authors as useful for individuals from high school through adult ages, so it is appropriate for this research study. It takes approximately 10 minutes to complete (Folkman & Lazarus, 1988). In this study, data from the WAYS were evaluated in three ways: total score on the 66 items (WAYS 66), total score on the 50 items (WAYS 50), and scores on the subscales. Reliability statistics for these scores in this study were comparable to those reported by Folkman and Lazarus (1988)" (Knapp, et al., 2013, p. 53).

3. Knapp et al. (2013) provided detailed information about the reliability of the STAI for previous studies and this study. The Cronbach alphas were very strong for this study at 0.92, indicating stronger reliability than previous studies with average Cronbach alphas at 0.86. The researchers also assessed the test-retest reliability of the scale with two participants, indicating that the scale is very stable (98%) with repeated measures. However, the discussion of the STAI validity is very limited. Researchers state only that the scale has been used in many studies over several years including families of the critically ill, similar to this study population. The scale is composed 40 items with 20 for state and 20 for trait anxiety, which indicates content validity and probably factor validity of this scale has been examined, but is not clearly discussed in this study. The measurement discussion would have been much stronger with coverage of types of validity (content validity and evidence of validity from contrasting groups, convergence, and/or divergence) and the readability level of the scale for this population. Stress is a complex concept that is difficult to measure with one scale and self-report on scales is also less valid than some other measures.

4. WAYS is identified as a questionnaire but is described as a 66-item Likert scale. The 8 coping subscales composed of 50 items indicate that content and probably factor validity of the scale have been examined, but are not clearly addressed in the study. The WAYS reliability is limited for previous research ranging from 0.61 to 0.79. It is unclear if these reliability values are for the total scale or for the subscales or both. With a reliability of 0.61, the scale has 61% reliability and 39% potential for error. The researchers did not report the reliability for the WAYS scale and subscales for this study, only that the reliability was comparable to other studies. Specific reliability values for the total scale and subscales for the participants in this study should be included in the research report. The researchers provided very limited information on the validity of the scale for previous studies or this study. The readability of this scale should be examined for this study population to ensure they have an understanding of the scale items. The two scales were pilot-tested on a sample of five family members but the details of the findings from the pilot are not discussed related to the instruments. The lower reliability values might have contributed to some of the nonsignificant findings for this scale.

5. Knapp et al. (2013) provided the following description of data collection:
"*Pilot Testing*
Two experts in family-centered critical care who were both doctorally prepared evaluated the content validity of the program. Three critical care nurses who worked in different unit pilot tested the computer-based educational component of the program. Minor adjustments to the program were made after the pilot testing. All instruments and procedures were pilot-tested on a sample of five family members prior to initiating the study.
Introduction of the Intervention… All nurses were invited to participate, and they were provided with information and the opportunity for open discussion, communication, and an exchange of ideas…
Data Collection Procedures
The study was conducted in three phases: pre-testing (control group), the intervention, and post-testing (intervention group).
Pre-testing
Pre-testing occurred prior to introduction of the intervention to gather data on the control group…
Intervention
The intervention was implemented over an 8 week period.
Post-testing
Eight weeks after implementation of the intervention, eligible family members were recruited to participate in the study following the same procedures as the pre-test phase. Data were collected for three months, from January to April, 2009" (Knapp et al., 2013, p. 54).
6. Knapp et al. (2013) provided a detailed description of the study intervention, the consistent implementation of the intervention by trained, doctorally prepared experts, and the pretesting and posttesting phase of collecting data with the STAI and WAYS scales. A strength of data collection is that the researchers conducted a pilot-test of the instruments and procedures in the study. The pilot was conducted on a sample of five family members with minor adjustments made to the program after this testing. However, no details are provided on the results of the pilot or the specific changes made in the study related to the pilot. Discussion of the pilot findings and changes made to the study would have strengthened the data collection section.

CHAPTER 11—UNDERSTANDING STATISTICS IN RESEARCH

EXERCISE 1: TERMS AND DEFINITIONS

1. o
2. c
3. f
4. n
5. e
6. m
7. b
8. j
9. a
10. g
11. l
12. d
13. h
14. i
15. k

EXERCISE 2: LINKING IDEAS

1. a. significant and predicted results
   b. nonsignificant results
   c. significant and unpredicted results
   d. mixed results
   e. unexpected results
2. You might have listed any of the following:
   a. findings
   b. significance of findings
   c. clinical importance of findings
   d. comparison of the findings from the current study to the findings from previous studies
   e. limitations
   f. conclusions
   g. generalization of findings
   h. implications for nursing
   i. recommendations for further study
3. You might have listed any of the following:
   a. management of missing data
   b. description of the sample and study variables
   c. reliability of measurement methods
   d. exploratory data analysis
   e. inferential statistical analysis
4. reduce and organize numerical data from a study to give it meaning
5. You might have listed any four of the following analysis techniques:
   a. Estimates of central tendency, such as mode, median, and mean
   b. Estimates of dispersion, such as range, variance, and standard deviation
   c. Examination of data to identify outliers
   d. Frequencies and percentages are calculated for nominal and ordinal data to determine the occurrence of demographic variables. For example, with a sample size of 220, the sample was 121 (55%) female and 99 (45%) male.
   e. Differences among groups are examined to demonstrate equivalence at the start of the study.

6. The normal curve is a symmetrical curve where the mean, median, and mode fall at the same point. See Figure 11-1 in Chapter 11 of your textbook, *Understanding Nursing Research*, 6th edition, for a drawing of the normal curve.
7. 95%
8. one-tailed test of significance
9. Type I error
10. ANOVA
11. mode
12. the group size
13. skewed or abnormally distributed curve
14. scatterplot
15. bivariate analysis

Linking Statistics with Analysis Techniques

1. b	6. a
2. e	7. h
3. j	8. g
4. c	9. d
5. f	10. i

Linking Levels of Measurement with Analysis Techniques

1. c	9. c
2. a	10. b and c
3. c	11. a
4. c	12. a and b
5. a and b	13. c
6. b	14. c
7. c	15. a and b
8. c	

Statements, Inferences, and Generalizations

1. d
2. b
3. a
4. c

Describing the Sample

1. Age in years
2. Associate Degree in Nursing (ADN)
3. 40-49 years
4. Standard deviation (SD) = 2.3
5. $95\% = \text{Mean} \pm 1.96(SD) = 15.5 \pm 1.96(2.3) = 15.5 \pm 4.51 = (10.99, 20.01)$

Measures of Central Tendency

1. 3.42
2. 3.10
3. The most frequent score or value in a distribution of scores. It is 3.00 in this example.
4. $\text{Mean} \pm SD = 3.42 + 0.76 = 4.18$ $3.42 - 0.76 = 2.66$ 2.66 to 4.18 or (2.66, 4.18)

Name That Statistical Analysis Technique!

1. d—Analysis of variance (ANOVA) testing for group differences with two or more groups; interval or ratio level data
2. a—Chi-square testing for differences; nominal level data
3. c—Pearson correlation is testing for relationships between variables; interval or ratio level data
4. b—*t*-test testing for differences between two groups; interval or ratio level data

Significance of Results

1. NS
2. *
3. *
4. NS
5. *

EXERCISE 3: WEB-BASED INFORMATION AND RESOURCES

1. a. Descriptive statistics included frequencies and percentages. Review the Data Collection and Analysis section in the article (Farrell & Shafiei, 2012, p. 1426).
   b. Inferential statistic included chi-squared tests to detect group differences.
   c. The study focused on estimating the prevalence of workplace aggression (WA) in nurses and midwives. "The prevalence of patient-initiated aggression and bullying among staff are clearly documented, which is in line with national (and international) trends. The data presented here suggest that the staff members are less worried by patient-initiated aggression compared to bullying from colleagues. Clearly, respondents wanted better training in WA. Also, they wanted effective enforcement of policies and management support when incidents arise" (Farrell & Shafiei, 2012, p. 1430).
   d. The researchers recommended qualitative studies to explore nurses' perceptions of what constitutes WA in all forms including patient-initiated aggression and bullying from colleagues. The effects of WA on bystanders also need to be examined. Studies to determine how to overcome WA need to be conducted.
2. a. Descriptive statistics included: frequencies, percentages, means, and standard deviations (see the Results section in Aronson et al., 2013, p. e125).
   b. Inferential statistics included Pearson r to examine relationships and t-tests to examine differences between pretest and posttest scores.

c. Limitations included the following: "The role-modeling intervention has been tested in only one academic setting with a small group of senior-level nursing students; therefore, the results cannot be generalized to other student populations....There is also a maturation threat inherent in the study [threat to internal validity, see Chapter 8]. It is not known whether student scores improved on the posttest, compared with the pretest because of increased clinical time during the students' capstone experience" (Aronson et al., 2013, p. e125). One group pretest–posttest design is not a strong design, and the study would have been strengthened by having both an experimental group and comparison group to determine the effect of the intervention (see Chapter 8 in your textbook, *Understanding Nursing Research*, 6th edition).

3. Wikipedia identifies several statistical resources on the following website: http://en.wikipedia.org/wiki/List_of_statistical_packages.
4. You can locate the Grove (2007) statistical workbook at the following URL: http://www.amazon.com/Statistics-Health-Care-Research-Practical/dp/141600226X.

EXERCISE 4: CONDUCTING CRITICAL APPRAISALS TO BUILD AN EVIDENCE-BASED PRACTICE

Bindler, Bindler, and Daratha (2013)

1. The subjects were originally selected as a single sample, but were then sorted into groups based on gender (male and female) and BMI percentile (<95th percentile and ≥95th percentile).
2. Link of variables, level of measurement, and descriptive data analysis techniques:

Demographic and study variables	Level of measurement	Descriptive analysis techniques
Age (months)	Ratio	Mean, standard deviation
Body mass index (BMI)	Ratio	Mean, standard deviation
Total cholesterol	Ratio	Mean, standard deviation
Systolic blood pressure	Ratio	Mean, standard deviation

3. Inferential statistics: Independent samples *t*-tests were conducted to examine group differences between males and females and the different BMI percentiles for the study variables. "Pearson correlation coefficients [r] were used to examine relationships between study variables and IR as measured by the log transformation of HOMA-IR... A multiple regression model was developed using the log transformation of HOMA-IR as the dependent variable and other study variables as potential predictor [or independent] variables" (Bindler et al., 2013, p. 22).
4. Mean HOMA-IR = 2.93 (see Table 1 in the Bindler article). The females had higher HOMA-IR values (3.26) than the males (2.49). Yes—females were significantly different from the males for the HOMA-IR values, as indicated by $p = 0.05$.
5. Waist circumference (cm) has the strongest correlation with HOMA-IR (see Table 3 in the article).
6. a. Yes, the correlation is statistically significant since $p < 0.001$ is smaller than the level of significance (alpha) that was set at 0.05 for the study.
   b. Yes. The correlation is clinically important since $r = .560$ is a strong correlation (see Chapter 11 in your textbook, *Understanding Nursing Research*, 6th edition) and explains 31.4% of the variance in HOMA-IR ($r^2 = .560^2 = 0.314 \times 100\% = 31.4\%$).
7. Waist circumference and triglycerides were used to predict HOMA-IR (see Table 4 in the Bindler article).
8. a. Yes. This result is statistically significant as indicated by $p < .001$), which is smaller than alpha (a) = 0.05.
   b. Yes. This result is clinically important since waist circumference and triglycerides explained 35% of the variance in HOMA-IR. Table 4 in the article identifies $R^2 = .35$ and percent of variance = $.35 \times 100\% = 35\%$.
9. Implications for pediatric nurses: "Pediatric nurses should always measure weight and height and then calculate BMI and BMI percentile for youth in all settings, being alert for those children and adolescents outside of the recommended weight for height parameters... For all youth, preventive interventions should be implemented... Waist circumference is a significant weight status measurement and should be evaluated with children displaying high BMI percentiles; additional data should include BP, dietary analysis, physical activity patterns, lipid panels, and glucose and insulin relationship. Youth identified with risk factors for IR and cardiometabolic outcomes need a 'downstream' approach with more intensive teaching and additional interventions to lower risk, measure progress toward outcomes, and continue monitoring their health status" (Bindler et al., 2013, p. 25).

Knapp, Sole, and Byers (2013)

1. Link of variables, level of measurement, and descriptive analysis techniques (see Table 1, Knapp et al., 2013, p. 54).

Demographic variables	Level of measurement	Descriptive analysis techniques
Relationship to patient	Nominal	Frequencies
Gender	Nominal	Frequencies
Ethnicity	Nominal	Frequencies
Patient age (years)	Ratio	Mean, range
Patient days in the SICU	Ratio	Mean, range

2. The anxiety levels were not significantly different between the groups as indicated by $p > 0.05$.
3. "*Distancing* and *accepting responsibility* subsets of coping were statistically significant between the two groups" (Knapp et al., 2013, p. 55).
4. a. Yes, this *t*-test is statistically significant since $p = .023$ and is smaller than the level of significance (alpha) that was set at 0.05 for the study.
   b. This result indicates significant improvement in the distancing coping score in the experimental group. The researchers state that "Higher scores were found in the experimental group, indicating improved coping in these two subsets after implementation of the [EPICS] Bundle" (Knapp et al., 2013, p. 55).
5. The researchers discussed several study limitations. "It was not possible to achieve the desired sample size in the allocated time period for the study… It was planned that the internet educational program would be mandatory for all staff members; however, management designated the program as optional. The program was completed by only 52 of 120 (43%) staff members in SICU… Several nurses did not fully support the intervention, and they may have influenced others… Education alone is not adequate for prompting a change within a nursing unit… Ideally, a control group and intervention group are tested at the same time. If this had been possible, the effect may have been greater" (Knapp et al., 2013, pp. 55-56).
6. Yes, the researchers did generalize their findings: "A firm foundation of information on how to decrease stress, and improve coping skills of families had been laid through this study, and it is anticipated it will promote evidence-based practice in the critical care setting. This foundation can also be expanded to other areas, such as emergency, rehabilitative services, or cardiovascular intensive care" (Knapp et al., 2013, p. 56). This generalization does not seem appropriate for this study based on the many limitations and the nonsignificant findings of the study. More studies are needed with larger sample size, stronger design, and greater intervention fidelity to determine the effectiveness of the EPICS Family Bundle on the stress and coping of families with members who are patients in the ICU following trauma.

CHAPTER 12—CRITICAL APPRAISAL OF QUANTITATIVE AND QUALITATIVE RESEARCH FOR NURSING PRACTICE

EXERCISE 1: TERMS AND DEFINITIONS

1. e
2. d
3. f
4. c
5. b
6. a

EXERCISE 2: LINKING IDEAS

1. strengths, weaknesses (limitations), meaning, and significance
2. You might include any three of the following:
   a. What are the major strengths of the study?
   b. What are the major weaknesses or limitations of the study?
   c. Are the findings of the study an accurate reflection of reality?
   d. What is the significance of the findings for nursing?
   e. Are the findings consistent with those of previous studies?
   (You can find these ideas in Box 12-1 in your textbook, *Understanding Nursing Research*, 6th edition.)
3. You might list any of the following or have other ideas:
   a. Critically appraise studies for class assignments.
   b. Critically appraise research to share the findings with other healthcare professionals.
   c. Read and critically appraise studies to solve a problem in practice.
   d. Critically appraise studies in a selected area and summarize the findings for use in practice.

   e. Critically appraise a proposed study to determine whether it is ethical to conduct in your clinical agency.
4. rights, informed consent
5. a. Purpose
   b. Qualitative approach
   c. Sample
   d. Key results

Understanding the Levels of Critical Appraisal for Quantitative Studies

1. b	11. a
2. b	12. b
3. a	13. b
4. c	14. c
5. b	15. b
6. c	16. b
7. a	17. b
8. a	18. a
9. b	19. b
10. c	20. c

Understanding the Levels of Critical Appraisal for Qualitative Studies

1. c	6. c
2. a	7. b
3. b	8. a
4. c	9. b
5. a	10. c

EXERCISE 3: WEB-BASED INFORMATION AND RESOURCES

1. The QSEN website for pre-licensure nursing students is: http://qsen.org/competencies/pre-licensure-ksas/.
2. The six QSEN Competency areas are:
   a. Patient-centered care
   b. Teamwork and collaboration
   c. Evidence-based practice (EBP)
   d. Quality improvement (QI)
   e. Safety
   f. Informatics
3. Evidence-based practice (EBP)
4. EBP Attitude: "Appreciate strengths and weaknesses of scientific bases [studies] for practice" (QSEN Website, 2013, p. 3).
5. EBP Skill: "Read original research and evidence reports related to area of practice" (QSEN Website, 2013, p.3).
6. The Magnet Recognition Program website is: http://www.nursecredentialing.org/Magnet.aspx.
7. Website to find agencies with Magnet status is: http://www.nursecredentialing.org/Magnet/FindaMagnetFacility.

EXERCISE 4: CONDUCTING CRITICAL APPRAISALS TO BUILD AN EVIDENCE-BASED PRACTICE

Conduct the critical appraisals of the three studies included in Appendices A, B, and C of this study guide. Review the answers to the critical appraisal exercises for Chapters 1 through 11 to assist yourself in these critical appraisals. Also, ask your instructor to clarify any questions that you might have.

CHAPTER 13—BUILDING AN EVIDENCE-BASED NURSING PRACTICE

EXERCISE 1: TERMS AND DEFINITIONS

1. m	8. f
2. k	9. d
3. h	10. i
4. b	11. g
5. e	12. c
6. j	13. a
7. l	14. n

EXERCISE 2: LINKING IDEAS

1. Evidence-based nursing practice promotes desired outcomes for patients, nurses, and healthcare agencies. You might have identified any of the following reasons (or others) for nurses to provide evidence-based practice:
   a. Improves quality of care
   b. Improves patient outcomes such as decreased signs and symptoms, improved functional status, improved physical and psychological health, prevention of illnesses, and increased promotion of health through implementation of healthy lifestyles
   c. Decreases recovery time
   d. Decreases need for healthcare services
   e. Decreases cost of care
   f. Improves work environment for nurses with increased productivity
   g. Increases access to care by providing different types of healthcare agencies and services with a variety of healthcare providers
   h. Increases patient satisfaction with care
   i. Important to meet accreditation requirements
   j. Important for a healthcare agency to achieve Magnet status
   k. Accomplishes a Quality and Safety Education for Nurses (QSEN) competency focused on promoting EBP
2. You might have identified any of the following:
   a. Read research journals in nursing and other healthcare disciplines.

b. Read clinical journals with a major focus on publishing research articles.
c. Use evidence-based websites such as the Agency for Healthcare Research and Quality and many others that communicate evidence-based guidelines and reference a variety of research publications. (See Table 13-1, Evidence-Based Practice Resources, in Chapter 13 of your textbook, *Understanding Nursing Research*, 6th edition.)
d. Attend professional nursing meetings and conferences.
e. Attend nursing research conferences.
f. Participate in collaborative groups of nurses and other health professionals that share research findings.
g. Note study findings reported on television and on the Internet.
h. Read research findings reported in newspapers and popular journals.

3. You might have identified any of the following:
   a. Nursing lacks the research evidence in certain areas for the implementation of evidence-based practice (EBP).
   b. There is a concern that research evidence generated based on population data might not transfer to the care of individual patients who respond in unique ways.
   c. The best research evidence is currently generated mainly from quantitative and outcomes research methodologies, and more work is needed to synthesize qualitative research and determine its contribution to EBP.
   d. The EBP movement might lead to the development of evidence-based guidelines that provide a narrow, specific approach that limits the care provided by healthcare providers.
   e. Healthcare agencies and administrators do not provide the resources to support the implementation of EBP by nurses.
4. You might have identified any of the following:
   a. EBP requires the synthesis of research evidence from randomized controlled trials, and these types of studies are limited in nursing.
   b. Researchers have found limited association between nursing interventions/processes and patient outcomes in acute care settings.
   c. There is significant variation in the methods to measure the effect of independent variables (nursing interventions) on patient outcomes.
   d. There is a need for additional studies to determine the effectiveness of nursing interventions.
   e. More replication studies are needed to strengthen the knowledge in significant areas of nursing practice.
   f. There is a need to identify areas where research evidence is needed for practice.
   g. Nurses need to be more active in conducting quality syntheses (systematic reviews, meta-analyses, meta-syntheses, and mixed-methods systematic reviews) of research evidence in selected areas.
5. a. Immediate use—using research-based intervention in practice exactly as it was developed.
   b. Reinvention—occurs when the research intervention is modified to meet the needs of a healthcare agency or nurses within the agency.
   c. Cognitive change—occurs when nurses incorporate research findings into their knowledge bases and use this information to defend a point, write agency protocols or policies, or develop a clinical paper for presentation.
6. Table 13-1 in Chapter 13 of your textbook, *Understanding Nursing Research*, 6th edition, provides several EBP resources.
   a. National Clearinghouse Guideline website (www.guideline.gov), which includes integrative reviews of research. This website was initiated by the Agency for Healthcare Research and Quality (AHRQ).
   b. Cochrane Library, which includes systematic reviews, meta-analyses, and integrative reviews of research to determine the best research evidence in selected practice areas. The Cochrane Reviews are available at http://www.cochrane.org/reviews/.
   c. Cochrane Nursing Care Field (CNCF) is included as part of the Cochrane Collaboration and supports the conduct, dissemination, and use of systemic reviews in nursing. The CNCF is available at http://cncf.cochrane.org/.
   d. The National Library of Health is located in the United Kingdom (UK); you can search for evidence-based sources using the following website: http://www.evidence.nhs.uk/.
   e. The National Institute for Health and Clinical Excellence (NICE) was organized in the United Kingdom to provide access to current EBP guidelines; it can be accessed at http://nice.org.uk/.
   f. The Joanna Briggs Institute is an international evidence-based organization in Australia that provides access to numerous evidence-based summaries. You can search the Joanna Briggs Institute website at http://joannabriggs.org/.

   g. The Nursing Reference Center (NRC) includes a collection of evidence-based care sheets that provide best practice for interventions and clinical conditions. The NRC requires a subscription, so check with your librarian.
   h. Meta-analyses and systematic reviews: Search CINAHL and MEDLINE for these types of research syntheses.
   i. Meta-syntheses and mixed-methods systematic reviews: Search CINAHL and MEDLINE for these types of research syntheses. You might also search for integrative reviews of research using these search engines.
7. The phases of the Stetler Model are:
   a. Phase I—Preparation
   b. Phase II—Validation
   c. Phase III—Comparative Evaluation/Decision Making
   d. Phase IV—Translation/Application
   e. Phase V—Evaluation
8. feasibility; current practice
9. a. Use research evidence in practice now.
   b. Consider using research knowledge in practice.
   c. Do not use the research findings in practice.
10. Agency for Healthcare Research and Quality
11. a. American Medical Association (AMA)
   b. American Association of Health Plans (AAHP), now call the American's Health Insurance Plans
12. Evidence-Based Practice
13. use of research evidence in practice or the use of evidence-based guidelines in practice

Application of the Phases of Stetler's Model

1. a	4. e
2. d	5. b
3. c	

Understanding Research Syntheses

1. b	6. a, b	11. d
2. d	7. c	12. a, b, c, d
3. c	8. a, b	13. a
4. a	9. b	14. b
5. a, b, c, d	10. c	15. c

Agency's Readiness for Evidence-Based Practice (EBP)

Obtain the answers to these questions by gathering information in the agency where you are doing your clinical hours this semester. Ask your faculty if these questions might be covered in class.

1. Review some of the protocols, algorithms, policies, and guidelines in the unit where you are doing clinical and note if the policies are documented with research sources. If these documents are without references, you cannot assume they are based on current research.
2. The policies, protocols, algorithms, and guidelines might be based on the knowledge and experience of the nurses developing them, but not documented with research references or evidence-based websites.
3. Are there nurses in the agency who are responsible for developing and revising policies, protocols, algorithms, and guidelines, and educating nurses to make the necessary changes in practice? Is there a team of nurses working toward meeting accreditation and Magnet status guidelines? These individuals are often the change agents in an agency and promote the use of evidence-based protocols, algorithms, policies, and guidelines in practice.
4. Ask the staff about access to a library in the agency. Do they have Internet access or hard copies of journals, and what are the names of the journals? Are these research journals or clinical journals with research articles? Do the nurses have access to evidence-based websites on the computers in the agency?
5. Ask nurses about the goal of EBP in their agency. What steps have been taken to promote EBP?
6. The healthcare agencies that currently have Magnet status can be viewed online at the American Nurses Credentialing Center (ANCC) website at http://www.nursecredentialing.org/Magnet/FindaMagnet-Facility.aspx (ANCC, 2014). Look on this website for the status of the agency. If the agency has Magnet status, how do they document the outcomes of care in their agency to maintain this status? If the agency is seeking Magnet status, where are they in the process of obtaining this designation? Having Magnet status indicates the agency has a commitment to EBP and excellence in nursing care.

EXERCISE 3: WEB-BASED INFORMATION AND RESOURCES

1. AHRQ National Guideline Clearinghouse website to search for evidence-based guidelines is http://www.guideline.gov/browse/by-topic.aspx.
2. Fall prevention in elderly guideline summary can be found at: http://www.guideline.gov/content.aspx?id=43933&search=fall+prevention.
3. ONS EBP guidelines for managing anxiety: https://www.ons.org/practice-resources/pep/anxiety
4. CNCF Cochran Reviews of Nursing Care website is: http://cncf.cochrane.org/cochrane-reviews-nursing-care.

5. NRC Patient Reference Center website is: http://www.ebscohost.com/nursing/products/patient-education-reference-center.
6. U.S. Preventive Services Task Force: Recommendations for Adults website is: http://www.uspreventiveservicestaskforce.org/adultrec.htm.
7. The website for the 2014 Hypertension Guidelines published by the *JAMA* can be found at http://jama.jamanetwork.com/article.aspx?articleid=1791497. Or you could have searched MEDLINE for this article.
8. The website for *Healthy People 2020* is http://www.healthypeople.gov/2020/default.aspx.
9. The website for Genomics can be found athttp://www.healthypeople.gov/2020/topicsobjectives2020/overview.aspx?topicid=15.

EXERCISE 4: CONDUCTING CRITICAL APPRAISALS TO BUILD AN EVIDENCE-BASED PRACTICE

1. The objective of the systematic review was "to examine the reported effectiveness of fall-prevention programs for older adults by reviewing randomized controlled trials from 2000 to 2009" (Choi & Hector, 2012, p. 188.e13). This objective was clearly and concisely presented and directed the methodology of the research synthesis.
2. The PICOS format was used to direct this research synthesis, as indicated by the following:
   - Population of older adults
   - Intervention of fall-prevention programs
   - Comparison of intervention and control groups
   - Outcomes were number of falls and fall rates
   - Study design was randomized controlled trials for 2000–2009
3. A detailed description of the rigorous literature search was provided on page 188.e14 of the article under the heading "Identification of Studies." The scientific and medical literature was searched using major biomedical electronic databases. "This rigorous literature examination selected articles in peer-reviewed journals published in English language, with full-text availability, targeting both men and women, in RCTs, with primary outcome measures as either the number of falls or the fall rate, with fall-intervention follow-up of a minimum of 5 months, and published from 2000 to 2009" (Choi & Hector, 2012, p. 188.e14).
4. A total of 287 studies were reviewed, and 17 studies were selected for the systematic review. The details of this selection process are presented in Figure 1, Flow Chart of Study Selection (Choi & Hector, 2012, p. 188.e15).
5. The quality of the 17 studies was determined by two blinded reviewers using the Downs and Black (DB) Checklist for Measuring Study Quality. In addition to the DB Checklist, the recommendations for reporting RCTs per Consolidated Standards of Reporting Trials (CONSORT) guidelines were applied (see Table 13-2 in your your textbook, *Understanding Nursing Research*, 6th edition, for the CONSORT guidelines for critically appraising and reporting RCTs).
6. Yes, a meta-analysis was conducted on the results from the 17 studies.
7. The authors developed a funnel plot of the 17 studies to examine for publication bias (see Figure 4 in the Choi and Hector article). They found evidence of bias in favor of publication of positive results in their meta-analysis.
8. Choi and Hector (2012) concluded that the fall-prevention programs conducted within the past 10 years were effective and had an overall fall reduction rate of 9%.

GOING BEYOND

1. Use the content in Chapter 13 of your textbook, *Understanding Nursing Research*, 6th edition, to implement an evidence-based practice project guided by Stetler's Model (textbook Fig. 13-6) or the Iowa Evidence-based Model (textbook Fig. 13-7).
2. Use the Grove Model in Figure 13-10 to direct the implementation of the evidence-based guidelines (Grove et al., 2015).

CHAPTER 14—INTRODUCTION TO OUTCOMES RESEARCH

EXERCISE 1: TERMS AND DEFINITIONS

1. f	7. e
2. h	8. l
3. g	9. k
4. a	10. c
5. d	11. j
6. i	12. b

EXERCISE 2: LINKING IDEAS

Key Ideas

1. Donabedian
2. a. Physical-psychological function
   b. Psychological function
   c. Social function
3. a. Structure: Nursing units, hospitals, clinics, or home health agencies
   b. Process: What care is provided or practice patterns of interventions provided patients. How

care is provided or practice style and standards of care delivered (clinical guidelines, critical paths, or care maps)
   c. Outcomes: Morbidity rates, mortality rates, length of stay in hospitals, complications from procedures, side effects of medications, medication errors, fall rates, infection rates, costs, or patient satisfaction
4. care by practitioners and other providers, care implemented by patient, and care received by community
5. nursing-sensitive outcomes
6. assessment, nursing diagnosis, nurse-initiated interventions
7. communication, case management, coordination of care, continuity, monitoring
8. outcome
9. a. Clinical guidelines
   b. Critical paths
   c. Care maps
10. funding opportunities; recently completed outcomes research
11. heterogeneous
12. You might have listed any of the following questions:
   a. What are the end results of patients' care (all care provided by all care providers)?
   b. What effect does nursing care (all care by all nurses) have on the end results of a patient's care?
   c. Are there some nursing acts that have no effect at all on outcomes or that actually cause harm?
   d. Can we measure and thus identify the end results of nursing care?
   e. How do we distinguish care provided by nurses from care provided by other professionals in examining patient outcomes?
   f. When do we measure the effects of care (end results) (e.g., change in symptoms, functioning, or quality of life): immediately after the care, when the patient is discharged, or much later?
13. a. Administrative
   b. Clinical
14. change; improvement
15. a. Are the results valid?
   b. What are the results?
   c. How can I apply the results to patient care?

Outcomes Research Methodologies

1. c
2. e
3. a
4. b
5. d

EXERCISE 3: WEB-BASED INFORMATION AND RESOURCES

1. Agency for Healthcare Research and Quality
   http://www.ahrq.gov/research/index.html
2. American Nurses Association
   http://www.nursingworld.org/
3. Collaborative Alliance for Nursing Outcomes California Database
   http://www.calnoc.org/
4. National Database of Nursing Quality Indicators
   http://www.nursingquality.org/
5. National Institute of Nursing Research
   http://www.ninr.nih.gov/
6. Nursing Interventions Classification
   http://www.nursing.uiowa.edu/cncce/nursing-interventions-classification-overview
7. National Quality Forum
   http://www.qualityforum.org/Home.aspx
8. Oncology Nursing Society
   http://www.ons.org/Research

EXERCISE 4: CONDUCTING CRITICAL APPRAISALS TO BUILD AN EVIDENCE-BASED PRACTICE

The critical appraisal was of the Galik and Resnick (2013) article found through your university library.

1. The Galik and Resnick (2013) article presents an outcomes study as indicated by the study title and purpose. "The purpose of this study was to describe the prevalence of psychotropic medication use among nursing home residents, and to explore the relationship of psychotropic medication use on physical and psychosocial outcomes" (Galik & Resnick, 2013, p. 244).
2. Physical outcomes measured were "specifically physical function and balance" (Galik & Resnick, 2013, p. 244). Muscle strength was also identified as measured on p. 246.

   Psychosocial outcomes measured were "specifically self-efficacy, outcome expectations for function, and quality of life" (Galik & Resnick, 2013, p. 244).
3. "This study was a **secondary data analysis** using data from a randomized controlled trial, the Res-Care Intervention Study (Resnick et al., 2009), combined with medication data abstracted from resident charts" (Galik & Resnick, 2013, p. 245).
4. The sample included **419 nursing home residents**. This is a large number of subjects and 69% (288) were prescribed at least one psychotropic medication, which was the focus of the study. The sample size was adequate for the study since the findings were significant for both physical and psychosocial outcomes. Therefore, no Type II error occurred.

5. The setting for the study was **12 nursing homes**. The use of data from multiple nursing homes strengthens the credibility of the findings and the ability to generalize the findings.
6. The researchers obtained **institutional review board (IRB) approval and either consent or assent** from the study participants. The consent process was strong as indicated by the following statement: "Participants completed their own consent if they passed the Evaluation to Sign Consent (Resnick et al., 2007). Those residents who were unable to pass the Evaluation to Sign Consent signed an assent to participate and the legally authorized representative provided proxy consents" (Galik & Resnick, 2013, pp. 245-246). Review the IRB approval and consent processes in Chapter 4 of your textbook, *Understanding Nursing Research*, 6th edition, to clarify any questions.
7. The **Dementia Quality of Life Instrument** was used to measure quality of life. This scale includes 29 items developed to measure self-esteem, positive affect, negative affect, feelings of belonging, and sense of aesthetics, which supports the content validity of the scale. The scale is appropriate for the study population since it was designed to be used with individuals who have mild to moderate dementia, which the study participants were assessed for using the Mini-Mental Status Exam (MMSE). The scale demonstrated internal consistency reliability with alpha coefficients ranging from 0.59 to 0.91. The scale also had "evidence of validity based on appropriate correlations with well-being and depression" (Galik & Resnick, 2013, p. 246).
8. The findings of the study are: "physical outcomes were significantly lower in residents receiving psychotropic medications ($F = 3.2, p = 0.01$) compared to those not receiving psychotropic medications. Psychosocial outcomes were significantly lower in those residents receiving psychotropic medications ($F = 2.0, p = 0.04$). The findings… suggest that residents receiving psychotropic medications may be less likely to engage in functional activities and experience decreased quality of life" (Galik & Resnick, 2013, p. 244).

APPENDIX

A Ågård et al. Study

Appendix A

Intensive and Critical Care Nursing (2012) **28**, 105–113

Available online at www.sciencedirect.com

SciVerse ScienceDirect

journal homepage: www.elsevier.com/iccn

Intensive and Critical Care Nursing

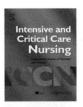

Struggling for independence: A grounded theory study on convalescence of ICU survivors 12 months post ICU discharge

A.S. Ågård[a,*], I. Egerod[b], E. Tønnesen[c], K. Lomborg[d]

[a] *Department of Anesthesiology and Intensive Care, Aarhus University Hospital, Brendstrupgårdsvej 100, DK-8200 Aarhus N, Denmark*

[b] *The University Hospitals Center for Nursing and Care Research, UCSF, Copenhagen University Hospital Rigshospitalet, Department 9701, Blegdamsvej 9, DK-2100 Copenhagen O, Denmark*

[c] *Department of Anesthesiology and Intensive Care, Aarhus University Hospital, Noerrebrogade 44, Building 21, DK-8000 Aarhus C, Denmark*

[d] *School of Public Health, Department of Nursing Science, Aarhus University, Hoegh-Guldbergs Gade 6A, Building 1633, DK-8000 Aarhus C, Denmark*

KEYWORDS
Intensive care;
Critical care;
Rehabilitation;
Family;
Caregivers;
Spouses;
Convalescence;
Recovery

Summary

Objectives: To explore and explain the challenges, concerns, and coping modalities in ICU-survivors living with a partner or spouse during the first 12 months post ICU discharge.

Design: Qualitative, longitudinal grounded theory study.

Settings: Five ICUs in Denmark, four general, one neurosurgical.

Methods: Thirty-five interviews with patients and their partners at three and 12 months post ICU discharge plus two group interviews with patients only and two with partners only.

Findings: The ICU survivors struggled for independence and focussed chiefly on 'recovering physical strength', 'regaining functional capacity', and 'resuming domestic roles'. The first year of recovery evolved in three phases characterised by training, perseverance and continued hope for recovery. The ICU survivors did not seem to worry about traumatic experiences. Rather, their focus was on a wide range of other aspects of getting well.

Conclusion: The study offers new insight into post-ICU convalescence emphasising patients' motivation for training to recover. The findings may contribute to defining the best supportive measures and timing of rehabilitation interventions in ICU and post ICU that may help ICU-survivors in their struggle for independence throughout recovery.

Introduction

Critical illness and admission to the intensive care unit (ICU) radically affects patients and their close relatives during hospitalisation and after discharge. Internationally, the long-term consequences of critical illness and ICU admission have been identified as an important professional issue

* Corresponding author. Tel.: +45 2162 5484; fax: +45 7845 1215.
E-mail addresses: anne.agard@reher-langberg.dk (A.S. Ågård), ie@ucsf.dk (I. Egerod), elsetoen@rm.dk (E. Tønnesen), kl@sygeplejevid.au.dk (K. Lomborg).

0964-3397/$ — see front matter © 2012 Elsevier Ltd. All rights reserved.
doi:10.1016/j.iccn.2012.01.008

(Angus and Carlet, 2003; Blackwood et al., 2011; Chaboyer et al., 2005; Dowdy et al., 2005).

After critical illness, ICU survivors often suffer from disease-specific sequelae, general physical and psychosocial problems requiring considerable efforts to regain pre-ICU functional level (NHS, National Institute for Health and Clinical Excellence 2009; Broomhead and Brett, 2002; Desai et al., 2011; Oeyen et al., 2010). Further, a substantial portion of ICU survivors experience cognitive impairment affecting memory, attention, and executive function (Desai et al., 2011). Deficits in these central functional areas may have important consequences for activities of daily living, health-care management and social functioning (Hopkins and Jackson, 2009). The prevalence of posttraumatic stress disorder is reported to be 5–63% (Jackson et al., 2007). For employed ICU survivors, the ability to return to work can be affected for months or indefinitely (Williams et al., 2010). The patients' health related quality of life has been reported to be generally lower than that of the background population in the first year after discharge (Chaboyer and Elliott, 2000; Dowdy et al., 2005), perhaps even longer (Ulvik et al., 2008).

The patients' close relatives are also affected by the adverse consequences of critical illness and its aftermath (Ågård and Harder, 2007; Linnarsson et al., 2010). As informal post-ICU caregivers, they may experience considerable lifestyle disruption and strain (Choi et al., 2011; Van Pelt et al., 2007).

In summary, recovery can be a strenuous time for both ICU survivors and their close relatives. Little is known, however, about the everyday concerns of ICU survivors and their cohabiting partners and the coping modalities employed to meet the challenges facing the couples. Better insight into these sparsely researched areas could provide health care staff with a stronger basis for preparing ICU survivors and their close relatives for post-ICU recovery.

The study is part of a larger project exploring the situation of ICU survivors and their cohabiting spouse or partner during the first 12 months following ICU discharge. The present study offers insight into some of the challenges facing ICU survivors and focusses chiefly on their concerns and coping modalities in the 12-months post ICU discharge. The next part of the project concerns the role of the partners during post ICU recovery and is in process. In the final part of the project we will address the concrete trajectories of patients and their partners.

Aim

The aim of the study was to explore the challenges facing ICU survivors with a cohabiting spouse or partner and explain patients' concerns and coping modalities during the first 12 months post ICU discharge.

Methods and material

Design and setting

The study was a qualitative, explorative, longitudinal study based on classic grounded theory (GT) methodology (Glaser, 1978; Glaser and Strauss, 1967) with a realist epistemological perspective (Lomborg and Kirkevold, 2003). Participants were from five Danish ICUs: four general ICUs (level 2 and 3) and one neurosurgical ICU (level 2) with 7–13 beds. The ICUs were situated at three university hospitals and one regional hospital. In 2009, the number of patients admitted to the five ICUs was 492–926 ranging from the smallest to the largest unit.

Participants and recruitment

Over a ten-month period, participants were recruited as a convenience sample from five ICUs. The heterogeneity of the ICU-population both pre and post ICU represents a challenge in ICU research (Herridge, 2007; Chaboyer and Elliott, 2000). Furthermore, when including relatives in post-ICU research, the type of relation is not always specified, although important differences have been found in the way the burden is experienced by the patient's partner, children, friends, parents, or other relatives (Foster and Chaboyer, 2003). To avoid some of the problems of heterogeneity, our inclusion criteria were quite narrow: (1) ICU survivors aged 25–70 years (people of working age), (2) intubation > 96 hours (to target the more severely ill patients) (Douglas and Daly, 2003), (3) patients with a cohabiting partner (potential primary caregiver after discharge), and (4) ability to communicate adequately in Danish.

To minimise the impact of prior illness on post-ICU recovery, we excluded patients with conditions that might have severely affected the patient's daily life prior to ICU admission (Orwelius et al., 2010). In addition to patients with major heart, lung, (e.g. Chronic obstructive pulmonary disease), or neurological disease, we also excluded patients with conditions such as depression, brain damage, schizophrenia, cancer, a recent history of drug/alcohol abuse prior to admission, or after attempted suicide. Finally, the patient was excluded if a pre-admission health status was missing in the hospital chart. Based on information from hospital charts, each potential participant was assessed for eligibility on a pragmatic basis by the first author.

Ethical considerations

After ethical and legal approval from the National Board of Health (J.nr. 7-604-04-2/158/EHE) and the Danish Data Protection Agency (J.nr. 2009-41-3022), we identified potential participants retrospectively from ward-based ICU databases and subsequent examination of hospital charts in five different ICUs. After careful selection, a total of 36 patients were identified consecutively by the first author. Before the initial contact we checked the hospital registers to make sure potential participants were alive. Subsequently, the patients and their partners were contacted by regular mail 10 weeks after ICU discharge and invited to participate in the study. Prospective participants were informed about the study verbally and in writing, the right to withdraw at any time, confidentiality and anonymity and asked to sign a letter of informed consent. A flow chart of the enrolment of patients and partners is provided in Fig. 1.

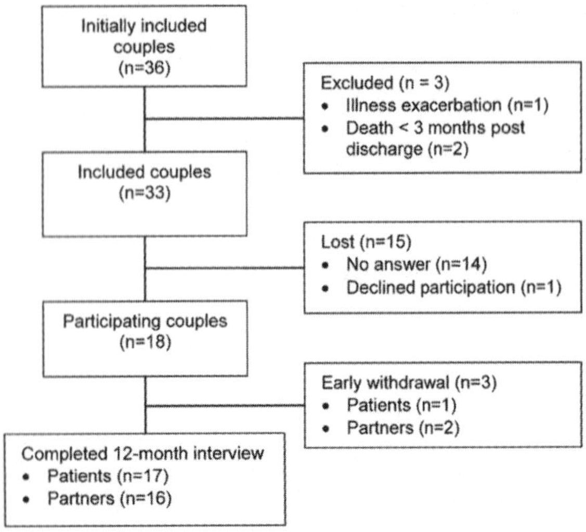

Figure 1 Patient and caregiver enrollment.

Data collection and analysis

Data consisted of dyad interviews with 18 patients and their partner at three ($n = 18 + 18$) and 12 ($n = 17 + 16$) months post ICU discharge. One couple and one partner withdrew from the study before the 12-month interview. The interviews took place in the couples' home or in a quiet room at the hospital. In addition to dyad interviews, we did two focus group interviews with patients only ($n = 3$ and $n = 7$) and two with partners only ($n = 2$ and $n = 7$), as there could be issues that the couples did not want to discuss openly (Svedlund and Axelsson, 2000; Hupcey, 1999). At the time of the group interviews some participants had been discharged 12–14 months ago, while others were discharged 3–4 months ago providing a wide range of patient experiences from different points in time after discharge. The group interviews were conducted somewhere between the three and 12-month interview rounds in meeting facilities at one of the hospitals.

The procedures of data collection, coding, memo writing, and analysis were performed concurrently using the constant comparative method central to GT methodology (Glaser and Strauss, 1967). During the initial three-month interviews, open coding was conducted and the core category "Struggling for independence" applied by the ICU-survivors to solve their main concerns was identified. As the analysis progressed, coding became more selective to identify further properties and dimensions of the emerging theory. The analytic perspective gradually evolved from a focus on particulars to a more general and conceptual level supported by written memos from the entire study period on the theoretical relationships between codes, categories, and concepts. As we focussed on recovery during the first 12 months after ICU discharge, we had to remain open to new insights throughout the entire process of data collection and analysis (Glaser, 1978). In the interviews participants elaborated on aspects from the time after ICU discharge giving examples from the entire recovery period. Writing memos helped us stay theoretically sensitive throughout the process of data collection and analysis as we were able to track the emergence of provisional ideas and compare those with later findings averting premature analytical conceptions (Glaser and Strauss, 1967). During the 12-month interviews, we coded both selectively and theoretically, while we further tested our ideas and looked for changes in concerns over time, while gradually saturating our substantive grounded theory.

The semi-structured interview guide was refined several times, as the interviews became more focussed in accordance with the principle of theoretical sampling and reflecting the emergence of our theory (Glaser and Strauss, 1967).

The 60–90 minute interviews were audio-taped and transcribed verbatim. The text version of the interviews provided the primary basis for the systematic coding and analysis. The first author conducted all interviews over a 19-month period in 2009–2010. The first and last authors contributed to the data analysis, which was supported by use of software package NVivo8.

Findings

Struggling for independence

During the first year of convalescence, the patients struggled for independence. The struggle evolved in three modalities: recovering physical strength, regaining functional capacity, and resuming domestic roles. These modalities followed a trajectory of three phases all characterised by training, perseverance, and continued hope for recovery (Table 2). Before we elaborate on the phases, in the following we present their context.

The context of post-ICU recovery

The Danish welfare system provides extensive financial and health care related security to Danish citizens. For a description of the Danish health care system, we refer to an official Danish website (The Ministry of the Interior and Health). Patient characteristics are provided in Table 1 to illustrate the context of everyday post-ICU recovery.

Patients were aged 35–70 years; 11 were men, 7 women. The ICU survivors, who were all generally in good health prior to critical illness, reported a wide range of complications in the first year after ICU discharge. The majority had experienced weight loss (5–25 kilos), fatigue, and loss of appetite. Two had persistent residual symptoms after critical illness polyneuropathy affecting their fine motor skills. Another patient had difficulty swallowing as a result of intubation. Depending on the ICU admission diagnosis, some of the patients also had various injuries causing reduced physical function (e.g. bone fractures) or impaired eyesight or hearing. One patient was initially quadriplegic, but partially recovered the use of his arms and legs.

Most of the patients with primary brain injuries or cerebral problems secondary to other conditions, e.g. hypoxia or septicaemia, reported cognitive symptoms such as reduced memory, concentration, or planning ability. Some patients with no known cerebral damage reported confusion or lack of initiative and reduced concentration or irritability in the initial period after ICU discharge and attributed these symptoms to their weak physical constitution in general. Two

Table 1 Patient characteristics in ICU and at 12 months post ICU discharge.

	Age	Sex	Type	LoS ICU	LoS Hosp.	LoS Rehab. facility	Th. physical	Th. neuropsych.	Th. private phys.	Sick leave F-T	Sick leave P-T	Pre-employment rate	Employment rate at 12 months
1	35	M	Trauma	11	12	—	12	—	—	353	0	37	20
2	39	F	Neuro	10	13	—	12	—	4	203	148	30	30
3	40	F	Cardiac	5	8	—	—	—	—	357	0	12	0
4	40	F	Gastric	67	8	106	20	13	—	251	0	37	16
5	40	M	Neuro	10	6	21	—	—	—	Ue	Ue	Ue	Ue
6	45	F	Pulmonary	73	47	119	28	—	—	92	107	37	12
7	50	M	Neuro	22	3	16	8	—	—	346	0	37	0
8	53	M	Trauma	11	9	—	—	—	—	154	120	37	37
9	55	F	Neuro	9	2	48	25	20	—	315	0	37	0
10	58	F	Pulmonary	10	37	—	8	—	—	90	0	15	15
11	60	M	Neuro	12	6	57	3	18	8	302	0	37	30
12	63	M	Trauma	11	42	—	34	—	—	323	0	37	0
13	64	M	Trauma	51	7	174	25	—	—	Ret	Ret	Ret	Ret
14	67	M	Cardiac	74	7	27	12	—	—	Ret	Ret	Ret	Ret
15	68	M	Cardiac	7	16	—	8	—	28	Ret	Ret	Ret	Ret
16	68	M	Trauma	21	3	55	8	—	—	Ret	Ret	Ret	Ret
17	70	M	Medical	8	63	15	5	—	—	Ret	Ret	Ret	Ret
18	70	F	Gastric	11	20	—	8	—	—	Ret	Ret	Ret	Ret

LoS = length of stay (days); Th. = therapy (weeks); F-T = full time (37 hours/week); P-T = part time (<37 hours/week); Ue = un-employed; Ret = retired.

ICU survivors recalled unpleasant hallucinations or unreal experiences, while two others remembered pleasant hallucinations. After a year none of the patients felt this was a problem.

Due to complications related to critical illness and hospitalisation, the patients still needed care upon their return home, leaving a substantial responsibility with the partner to provide the care needed, and most of the patients reported experiencing a renewed feeling of connectedness with their partner and family. Besides their everyday household activities and general support, the partners assisted with, e.g. meals, medications, personal hygiene, planning, social activities, and transportation to the hospital or general practitioner. After 12 months, three out of 11 patients had resumed their pre-ICU employment rate.

For the ICU survivors the 12-month post-ICU period of recovery was generally characterised by hope for further recovery. Some of the patients experienced progress or even recovery in most areas, while others still struggled with residual complications 12 months post-ICU discharge.

Recovering physical strength

Essential to the patients' struggle for independence was their effort to re-establish premorbid physical strength, which required months of training partly in hospital or in a rehabilitation facility and partly in community-based programmes (Table 1). Most of the participants had lost weight and muscular strength during hospitalisation. The resulting physical weakness required a lot of effort to regain normal physical strength for everyday activities such as getting out of bed, getting up from a chair, showering, dressing, climbing stairs, and moving about in the house or outside. This is summarised by an elderly male describing his situation prior to transfer to rehabilitation:

> "Then I had to try to get up with a walker and I just couldn't. I couldn't even hold my head. I wasn't able to do anything."
>
> (ID no. 14, male, 67 years)

Later, exercise was directed towards recovering physical strength for short walks outside, shopping, gardening, etc. gradually expanding the range of activities. Even after substantial training for a year, not all participants had returned to their pre-ICU level of physical strength and activity. An elderly male explained during the 12-month interview:

> "The most difficult bit was . . . I felt it took forever before I regained my strength. I just deposited my physical strength at the hospital and I still feel it. I mean, I don't feel I am up to my usual strength yet. I need an afternoon nap, sometimes two. I feel that I need more strength to open the lid of a jar of jam. I was actually quite strong before I got sick."
>
> (ID no. 15, male, 68 years)

During the first months after ICU discharge, the training activities combined with frequent hospital appointments often entailed a tight schedule for the patients leaving little energy for other activities such as interaction with friends and family during the week.

Regaining functional capacity

While gradually recovering their physical strength, the patients simultaneously tried to regain functional capacity allowing them to perform pre-ICU everyday activities. As a patient stated at the 12 month interview: "*Happiness is doing things yourself*" (ID no. 9).

Regaining functional capacity involved developing new ways of performing all sorts of activities to compensate for possible physical or cognitive shortcomings whether temporary or permanent. If the patients were not fully capable of performing a specific activity, they would try again later or find a different way of performing the activity, or the partner would assist them to complete the activity or take over. To illustrate the many accounts of this type of resourcefulness, a patient explained during the 12-month interview:

> "In the beginning when I came home and wanted to go upstairs, I sat on my behind and went up and down the stairs. It took a while before I could get around."
>
> (ID no. 6, female, 45 years)

Patients with cognitive impairment had to relearn performing basic activities such as dressing, personal hygiene, keeping track of things, cooking, cleaning, etc. Even if the cognitive deficits had a major impact on their everyday capabilities, most often the patients failed to report their difficulties, suggesting perhaps inability to acknowledge, accept, or comprehend the gravity of their situation. If the patients lacked this insight, the partner would recall situations where they had supported the patient in activities requiring these skills.

Typically, the partners were involved in situations where the patient's functional capacity was inadequate, such as actively helping with a specific activity or by rearranging things in and around the house.

As the patients gradually recovered basic functions during recovery, their goals shifted towards practicing functions at a more complex and complicated level such as planning, organising, shopping, driving a car again, or perhaps returning to work. Regaining their functional capacity, the ICU survivors were pleased as they gradually became independent of the health care system or the social system.

Resuming domestic roles

Resuming domestic roles was central to the patients' struggle for independence. After their illness, the patients were weak and unable to worry about the extent of help from their partners. Later, they became increasingly aware of their changed roles in their relationship with their partner. During recovery the patients gradually attempted to reduce their dependency and the burden on their spouse. As a patient said at the 12-month interview:

> "I probably went too far. I mean, I was at home and tried to arrange that my husband didn't need to come home and do things. But then I was tired and couldn't handle it anyway."
>
> (ID no. 2, female, 40 years)

Table 2 The three phases in patients' coping modalities during the first year of post-ICU recovery.

	Feeling one's way	Getting a grip	Maintaining and refining
Recovering physical strength	Training to recover basic physical strength for performing basic everyday indoor activities with little idea of the effort needed to recover premorbid physical strength	Training to recover additional physical strength for performing more physically demanding tasks in and around the home while gradually realising the extent of the physical training needed to recover	Continued efforts to recover further physical strength or maintain their level of strength while gradually expanding the range of the patients' physical activities
Regaining functional capacity	Trying to perform basic everyday activities alternating with periods of rest or sleep	Gradually developing new ways of performing all sorts of activities to compensate for temporary or permanent disabilities	Practicing functions at a progressively more complex and complicated level both physically and psychosocially
Resuming domestic roles	Being relatively dependent on help from the partner and accepting the help provided often without considering the extent of the help	Testing the range of their functional capability and still leaning to some extent on assistance from the partner while being increasingly aware of the help provided	Gradually becoming independent of assistance while actively freeing themselves more and more of their partner's help and expanding their territory in the relationship

The patients had an active role in minimising their partner's help. Generally, the patients felt their partner was there for them in a helpful way. On the other hand, as they gradually recovered, several patients mentioned incidents where they had actively confronted their partner telling them to stop their help or advice. The patients were annoyed by the partner's interference, when they felt capable of performing a certain activity, big or small. They gradually expanded their territory in the interactions with their partner. At the 12-month interview one patient said:

> "But this is also something we have had to deal with, from me being the one that was protected in all situations in the best possible way, to my husband who had a hard time accepting that now I wanted to do things myself. I couldn't . . . I felt overprotected; I was able to unpack my own suitcase. We went on and on about this. It was simply that our roles had to return to normal, because I was almost myself again."
>
> (ID no. 9, female, 55 years)

When asked about the characteristics of this evolving process, the participants described it as an intuitive trial-and-error approach continuously testing their capabilities while leaning to some extent on assistance from their partner. The patients wanted to avoid being a burden to others: "*It sucks knowing that I am a burden*" (Patient ID no. 3 at group interview). This affected recovery in various ways as illustrated in the following quote:

> "You know what, I don't want to go home and have my wife help me get to bed and help me go to the bathroom – and if I fall – I just don't want to be a burden to her. That's it! When I can walk again it will be different."
>
> (ID no. 13, male, 64 years, at three months)

Three phases

The first year of recovery evolved in three phases all characterized by training, perseverance, and continued hope of recovery. A summarising description of the phases is provided in Table 2.

Training, perseverance, and continued hope for recovery were the vehicles that moved the process of struggling for independence forward taking the patient from one phase to another. Physical strength was a prerequisite for the patients' effort to regain functional capacity, and with increased functioning the patients resumed their domestic roles. Improving any aspect of functional level increased the patients' momentum to keep on struggling for independence. Through statements like: "*Keep going*", "*Be patient*", "*Hang in there*" (physical training), or "*Don't give up*" they all emphasised the need to continue even if things were tough. The participants provided rich descriptions of the feeling of reward when progress was made. In general, whether they had more or fewer complications, the patients all expressed a strong motivation and resourcefulness to regain the best possible functional level physically as well as psychosocially, and 12 months post ICU there was still hope for further recovery. The patients acknowledged the importance of their partners' efforts moving the process of recovery forward when they themselves lost their resolve.

Discussion

The primary finding of the study was that the study patients did not seem to worry about traumatic experiences or psychological complications. Instead, their focus was on overcoming everyday physical and functional challenges, and the patients showed resourcefulness.

Studies on psychosocial complications after critical illness, e.g. posttraumatic stress, depression, or anxiety, have shown that these conditions are common amongst ICU-survivors (Oeyen et al., 2010; Davydow et al., 2008; Desai et al., 2011). Hence, we were surprised to learn that the ICU survivors in our study did not seem to worry about traumatic experiences or memories of being in intensive care or from the incident that initially caused their illness. Instead, they focussed on other aspects of recovery that are common amongst non-intensive care patients. For ethical reasons, we were unable to ask non-participants about their reasons for declining, and consequently we can only speculate about this. The patients were invited to participate in the study 10 weeks post ICU-discharge when the prospects for recovery were still unclear to most of them. In the study group, however, both ICU survivors struggling with major and minor complications were represented, suggesting that they did not influence the decision to participate.

There may be various reasons why the patients appeared less psychologically traumatised than earlier studies indicate. First, the patients did not seem to have symptoms of trauma. At three and 12 months, most of the patients had no recollection of their time in ICU. They were generally grateful to have survived and appreciated the lifesaving treatment and care provided by professionals who they also failed to recall. The patients did not look back to re-live their ICU experiences; they looked to the future and concentrated on regaining the abilities they had lost. This is in conflict with ICU literature describing the trauma of intensive care but might to some extent be explained by looking at the context of our study. The participants were recruited from ICUs representing a new paradigm in intensive care encouraging less sedation, shorter duration of mechanical ventilation, early mobilisation, awareness of delirium, and more family collaboration (Egerod, 2009). Consequently, less negative patient experiences could be reflections of improvements in intensive care.

There are indications that the focus on physical recovery precedes the focus on psychological recovery. Therefore, if the follow-up period had extended to more than 12 months, a tendency towards more emotional problems might be found (Oeyen et al., 2010). Therefore, we encourage follow-up studies beyond 18 or 24 months post ICU discharge.

Generally, the patients did not feel their experiences had been traumatising. On the other hand, a few patients had problems with concentration or increased irritability, which may be diffuse symptoms of depression or post-traumatic stress disorder (American Psychiatric Association (APA), 2006). As these conditions often associated with post-ICU recovery can only be properly detected through systematic screening, we were unable to establish if the diffuse symptoms mentioned could be indicators of psychiatric conditions.

Another explanation could be that the patients in our study all had their spouses by their side supporting them in hospital and at home. Studies show that close relatives help patients understand what happened in ICU and help them come to terms with the illness experience as a part of their recovery (Egerod et al., 2011). The patients' family has been described as a lifeline for the patient in ICU (Bergbom and Askwall, 2000) as well as after discharge, and their role in post-ICU recovery is an important area for future research (Paul and Rattray, 2008).

The study participants were generally in good health before their critical illness and therefore had a robust starting point for recovery. This could be another reason why they did not seem traumatised. Orwelius and colleagues found, that previously healthy ICU patients had a health-related quality of life (HQOL) after ICU almost identical to that of a group of non-hospitalised citizens that were not entirely healthy, but had no history of critical illness or admission to ICU (Orwelius et al., 2010). The authors reported that ICU-related factors such as APACHE II score, length of stay in ICU, and ventilator time were not associated with HQOL, whereas pre-existing disease prior to ICU admission accounted for most of the reduction in HQOL in ICU survivors (ibid). Consequently, future studies of post-ICU recovery should look at pre-existing disease.

The study patients suffered a range of physical and psychosocial sequelae with varying impact on their everyday lives. The reported complications were consistent with those described in the literature (Desai et al., 2011). The patients' main concern across the reported range of complications was to overcome the obstacles on their road to recovery. Their main object was similar to the goals of recovery for patients suffering from spinal cord injuries (Angel, 2010) or other less life-threatening illnesses (Sigurgeirsdottir and Halldorsdottir, 2008). Elements of the three phases of post-ICU recovery were found in recovery after spinal cord injury (Angel, 2009). The ICU recovery phases were also similar to aspects of theories of crisis and coping in general (Cullberg, 1993), indicating universal phenomena of recovery.

The quality of life of some of the study participants was at times significantly reduced, which is not surprising considering the gravity of their illness and the efforts needed to recover. Even so, patients also reported experiencing new qualities in life such as renewed feelings of connectedness with their partner and family and gratitude for being alive that seemed to fundamentally influence their recovery. We did not systematically evaluate quality of life, but we were encouraged to learn that some patients also had positive experiences after critical illness, even if they suffered from physical or cognitive sequelae. These aspects of post-ICU recovery would probably have remained invisible in conventional quality of life studies.

When researchers in the past have discussed the difficulties of ICU survivors, they may have neglected to describe less spectacular reactions to intensive care, thus leaving a gap in the current body of knowledge. To paint a more complete picture of ICU-recovery, we suggest to further integrate more general aspects of rehabilitation shared with non-ICU patients and to also describe possible positive perspectives, as in a recent study (Samuelson, 2011), without neglecting the challenges facing patients and their families in ICU and after discharge.

Our study shows, that in spite of various problems after critical illness, patients and their partners could be resourceful. Similar results were found in a group of patients with spinal cord injuries (Angel, 2010). As there is still some uncertainty as to the effects of existing post-ICU follow-up programmes (Cuthbertson et al., 2009) involving the resources and experiences of ex-patients and relatives in

Appendix A

community-based support groups could be a promising supplement to existing hospital based follow-up programmes (Peskett and Gibb, 2009).

In GT-methodology, the criteria for critically appraising a theory are whether it 'fits', 'works', is 'relevant' and 'modifiable' (Glaser, 1978; Lomborg and Kirkevold, 2003). As we carefully adhered to the analytic strategies of the methodology, we believe the theory fits the data from which it evolved offering a coherent theory on the patients' main concern and coping modalities employed to overcome post-ICU challenges. In spite of narrow criteria for inclusion, the characteristics of our study participants varied considerably. Even so, we found concurrent patterns in the patients' main concerns and behaviour increasing the scope of the theory and adding to the workability of the theory to explain, predict, and interpret what is happening in post-ICU recovery. We believe the theory is relevant to health care providers striving to support ICU survivors in the first year of recovery. As it also seems to imply some universal elements of recovery, we believe it also could be modified for groups of non-intensive care patients.

Long-term ICU rehabilitation is a growing field of interest to health care professionals and researchers. To enhance our current understanding of post-ICU recovery, we suggest seeking further inspiration and perspectives from other medical specialties including illnesses that are less life-threatening and in areas with more experience in rehabilitation, e.g. occupational therapy or physiotherapy. Increased awareness amongst ICU-staff of post-ICU patients' motivation for training could contribute to promoting early mobilisation in ICU. Besides reducing patients' physical impairment, early mobilisation could also contribute to instilling hope and empowering patients in the early process of recovery.

As more patients survive critical illness and face the challenges of recovery, survivorship could be the defining challenge in critical care encouraging new approaches to treatment and care (Iwashyna, 2010). We suggest that qualitative research approaches are applied to gain further insight into the challenges facing patients in ICU and after discharge. Furthermore, in line with the principles of family-centred care in ICU (Davidson et al., 2007), future research on the role of patients' close relatives after ICU discharge is an important issue that could yield new insights providing a more holistic basis for the continued efforts of health care professionals and researchers to improve treatment and care.

Conclusion

In this grounded theory study of recovery 12 months post ICU, the patients struggled for independence and focussed chiefly on exercising to recover physical strength, regaining functional capacity and resuming domestic roles. The first year of recovery evolved in three phases characterised by training, perseverance, and continued hope of recovery. The patients in our study did not verbalise traumatic experiences or recollections from intensive care. Instead, their focus was on recovery similar to that of non-intensive care patients.

The findings from this qualitative study offer new insights into the trajectories of ICU survivors and their concerns after critical illness complementing our current understanding of post-ICU recovery. The findings may contribute to defining the best supportive measures and timing for post-ICU rehabilitation that may help ICU survivors in their struggle for independence throughout recovery.

Conflict of interest statement

The authors and the funders have no financial or personal relationships that could inappropriately influence this work.

Acknowledgements

We are grateful to the participating patients, spouses, and partners for sharing their experiences of life after ICU. Also, we thank the ICU nurses and administrative staff who facilitated the collection of data. Thanks also to Janet Mikkelsen, Department of Public Health, Aarhus University for help in editing the manuscript language. The study was supported by grants from The Novo Nordisk Foundation, The Health Insurance Foundation, The Danish Nurses' Organisation, Aarhus University Hospital, The Aase and Ejnar Danielsen Foundation, The Lundbeck Foundation and The Central Jutland Region.

Contributors: ASÅ, KL, ET, IE contributed in the conception and design of the study; ASÅ, KL in drafting the manuscript; ASÅ, KL, ET, IE in improving the manuscript; the final approval was made by ASÅ.

References

Ågård AS, Harder I. Relatives' experiences in intensive care—finding a place in a world of uncertainty. Intensive Crit Care Nurs 2007;23(3):170–7.

APA practice guidelines for the treatment of psychiatric disorders: comprehensive guidelines and guideline watches; practice guideline for the treatment of patients with acute stress disorder and posttraumatic stress disorder. American Psychiatric Publishing, Inc.; 2006. Available from: http://psychiatryonline.org/content.aspx?bookid=28&sectionid=1670530#52640 [Accessed 01/05/2012].

Angel S. Vulnerable, but strong: the spinal cord-injured patient during rehabilitation. Int J Qual Stud Health Well-being 2010;5(October (3)), 10.3402/qhw.v5i3.5145.

Angel S. Getting on with life following a spinal cord injury: regaining meaning through six phases. Int J Qual Stud Health Well-being 2009;4(1):39–50.

Angus DC, Carlet J, editors. Surviving intensive care. Heidelberg: Springer-Verlag Berlin; 2003.

Bergbom I, Askwall A. The nearest and dearest: a lifeline for ICU patients. Intensive Crit Care Nurs 2000;16(6):384–95, 12//;.

Blackwood B, Albarran JW, Latour JM. Research priorities of adult intensive care nurses in 20 European countries: a Delphi study. J Adv Nurs 2011;67(March (3)):550–62.

Broomhead LR, Brett SJ. Clinical review: intensive care follow-up--what has it told us? Crit Care 2002;6(October (5)):411–7.

Chaboyer W, James H, Kendall M. Transitional care after the intensive care unit: current trends and future directions. Crit Care Nurse 2005;25(June (3)):16.

Chaboyer W, Elliott D. Health-related quality of life of ICU survivors: review of the literature. Intensive Crit Care Nurs 2000;16(April (2)):88–97.

Choi J, Donahoe MP, Zullo TG, Hoffman LA. Caregivers of the chronically critically ill after discharge from the intensive care unit: six months' experience. Am J Crit Care 2011;20(January (1)):12–22.

Cullberg J. Krise og udvikling: en psykoanalytisk og socialpsykiatrisk studie [Crisis and development: a psychoanalytical and social psychiatric study]. 4. udgave ed. Kbh.: Hans Reitzel; 1993.

Cuthbertson BH, Rattray J, Campbell MK, Gager M, Roughton S, Smith A, et al. The PRaCTICaL study of nurse led, intensive care follow-up programmes for improving long term outcomes from critical illness: a pragmatic randomised controlled trial. BMJ 2009;339(October):b3723.

Davidson JE, Powers K, Hedayat KM, Tieszen M, Kon AA, Shepard E, et al. Clinical practice guidelines for support of the family in the patient-centered intensive care unit: American college of critical care medicine task force 2004–2005. Crit Care Med 2007;35(2):605–22.

Davydow DS, Gifford JM, Desai SV, Needham DM, Bienvenu OJ. Posttraumatic stress disorder in general intensive care unit survivors: a systematic review. Gen Hosp Psychiatry 2008;30(September–October (5)):421–34.

Desai SV, Law TJ, Needham DM. Long-term complications of critical care. Crit Care Med 2011;39(February (2)):371–9.

Douglas SL, Daly BJ. Caregivers of long-term ventilator patients: physical and psychological outcomes. Chest 2003;123(April (4)):1073–81.

Dowdy DW, Eid MP, Sedrakyan A, Mendez-Tellez PA, Pronovost PJ, Herridge MS, et al. Quality of life in adult survivors of critical illness: a systematic review of the literature. Intensive Care Med 2005;31(May (5)):611–20.

Egerod I. Cultural changes in ICU sedation management. Qual Health Res 2009;19(May (5)):687–96.

Egerod I, Christensen D, Schwartz-Nielsen KH, Ågård AS. Constructing the illness narrative: a grounded theory exploring patients' and relatives' use of intensive care diaries. Crit Care Med 2011;39(May (8)):1922–8.

Foster M, Chaboyer W. Family carers of ICU survivors: a survey of the burden they experience. Scand J Caring Sci 2003;17(3):205–14.

Glaser BG. Theoretical sensitivity. Advances in the methodology of grounded theory. Mill Valley, CA: Sociology Press; 1978.

Glaser BG, Strauss AL. The discovery of grounded theory: strategies for qualitative research. Hawthorne, New York: Aldine de Gruyter; 1967.

Herridge MS. Long-term outcomes after critical illness: past, present, future. Curr Opin Crit Care 2007;13(October (5)):473–5.

Hopkins RO, Jackson JC. Short- and long-term cognitive outcomes in intensive care unit survivors. Clin Chest Med 2009;30(March (1)):143–53, ix.

Hupcey JE. Looking out for the patient and ourselves—the process of family integration into the ICU. J Clin Nurs 1999;8(3):253–62.

Iwashyna TJ. Survivorship will be the defining challenge of critical care in the 21st century. Ann Intern Med 2010;153(August (3)):204–5.

Jackson JC, Hart RP, Gordon SM, Hopkins RO, Girard TD, Ely EW. Post-traumatic stress disorder and post-traumatic stress symptoms following critical illness in medical intensive care unit patients: assessing the magnitude of the problem. Crit Care 2007;11(1):R27.

Linnarsson JR, Bubini J, Perseius KI. Review: a meta-synthesis of qualitative research into needs and experiences of significant others to critically ill or injured patients. J Clin Nurs 2010;19(21–22):3102–11.

Lomborg K, Kirkevold M. Truth and validity in grounded theory—a reconsidered realist interpretation of the criteria: fit, work, relevance and modifiability. Nurs Philos 2003;4:189–200.

NHS, National Institute for health and Clinical Excellence: rehabilitation after critical illness; 2009. Available from: www.nice.org.uk/CG83 [Accessed 01/05/2012].

Oeyen SG, Vandijck DM, Benoit DD, Annemans L, Decruyenaere JM. Quality of life after intensive care: a systematic review of the literature. Crit Care Med 2010;38(December (12)):2386–400.

Orwelius L, Nordlund A, Nordlund P, Simonsson E, Backman C, Samuelsson A, et al. Pre-existing disease: the most important factor for health related quality of life long-term after critical illness: a prospective, longitudinal, multicentre trial. Crit Care 2010;14(April (2)):R67.

Paul F, Rattray J. Short- and long-term impact of critical illness on relatives: literature review. J Adv Nurs 2008;62(3):276–92.

Peskett M, Gibb P. Developing and setting up a patient and relatives intensive care support group. Nurs Crit Care 2009;14(January–February (1)):4–10.

Samuelson KAM. Unpleasant and pleasant memories of intensive care in adult mechanically ventilated patients—findings from 250 interviews. Intensive Crit Care Nurs 2011;27(2): 76–84.

Sigurgeirsdottir J, Halldorsdottir S. Existential struggle and self-reported needs of patients in rehabilitation. J Adv Nurs 2008;61(4):384–92.

Svedlund M, Axelsson I. Acute myocardial infarction in middle-aged women: narrations from the patients and their partners during rehabilitation. Intensive Crit Care Nurs 2000;16(August (4)):256–65.

The Ministry of the Interior and Health: Health Care in Denmark. Available from: http://www.sum.dk/Aktuelt/Publikationer/Publikationer/UK_Healthcare_in_DK.aspx [Accessed 01/05/2012].

Ulvik A, Kvale R, Wentzel-Larsen T, Flaatten H. Quality of life 2–7 years after major trauma. Acta Anaesthesiol Scand 2008;52(February (2)):195–201.

Van Pelt DC, Milbrandt EB, Qin L, Weissfeld LA, Rotondi AJ, Schulz R, et al. Informal caregiver burden among survivors of prolonged mechanical ventilation. Am J Respir Crit Care Med 2007;175(January (2)):167–73.

Williams TA, Leslie GD, Brearley L, Dobb GJ. Healthcare utilisation among patients discharged from hospital after intensive care. Anaesth Intensive Care 2010;38(4):732–9.

APPENDIX

B Bindler et al. Study

Journal of Pediatric Nursing (2013) **28**, 20–27

ELSEVIER

Appendix B

Biological Correlates and Predictors of Insulin Resistance Among Early Adolescents

Ross J. Bindler BS, PharmD Candidate [a], Ruth C. Bindler RNC, PhD [b,*], Kenneth B. Daratha PhD [b]

[a]*Washington State University, College of Pharmacy, Spokane, WA*
[b]*Washington State University, College of Nursing, Spokane, WA*

Key words:
Insulin resistance;
Hyperinsulinemia;
Obesity;
Adolescent;
Diabetes mellitus Type 2

Abnormal glucose metabolism is associated with obesity, insulin resistance (IR), and Type 2 diabetes mellitus. The purposes of this study were to describe anthropometric and laboratory markers of adolescents, examine correlates of IR, and test ability of anthropometric and laboratory markers to predict risk of exhibiting IR. A total of 150 early adolescents participated. Participants with obesity had increased IR, high-sensitivity C-reactive protein, triglycerides, and blood pressure. Waist circumference and triglycerides were predictive of IR. Multiple risk factors compound and lead to long-term health consequences among youth. Nurses can evaluate these factors to identify IR.

PREVALENCE OF OBESITY is at historic high levels among youth; for example, worldwide, obesity has doubled, and in developed countries, the numbers of youth who are overweight or obese have tripled in the last three decades (Ogden et al., 2006; World Health Organization, 2011). Insulin resistance (IR) is associated with obesity and abnormal glucose metabolism and transport and can lead to a prediabetic state (Lee, Okumura, Davis, Herman, & Gurney, 2006; Li, Ford, Huang, Sun, & Goodman, 2009; Liu et al., 2009; Monzavi et al., 2006). In IR, muscle, fat, and liver cells cannot respond adequately to insulin, and therefore, increased insulin production occurs; high levels of both serum glucose and insulin are present at the same time (National Diabetes Information Clearinghouse, 2008).

Review of Literature, Purpose, and Study Aims

Obesity and IR in youth are associated with increased prevalence of a variety of cardiometabolic risk factors and promotion of fat mass development. Several body measurements, for example, waist circumference and waist to hip ratio, are correlated with IR (Bitsori, Linardakis, Tabakaki, & Kafatos, 2009; Cossio et al., 2009). Cardiometabolic markers such as lipid and triglyceride levels are also related to IR in adolescence (Kim-Dorner, Deuster, Zeno, Remaley, & Poth, 2010), and biological markers of inflammation increase when IR is present (Park, Steffes, Lee, Himes, & Jacobs, 2009). Some youth with IR develop Type 2 diabetes mellitus (T2D); in fact, up to 45% of youth newly diagnosed with diabetes now have Type 2 disease, a phenomenon nearly unheard of in youth just a few years ago (Centers for Disease Control and Prevention [CDC], 2010; Lee et al., 2006; Shah et al., 2009). Youth with obesity and polycystic ovary syndrome are more likely to have IR, T2D, and impaired glucose tolerance (Nur, Newman, & Siqueira, 2009). Youth with overweight, hyperlipidemia, and IR should be evaluated for nonalcoholic fatty liver disease (Mager, Ling, & Roberts, 2008). Body mass index (BMI) and waist circumference both predict IR in children at time of school entry, and females are more likely than males to demonstrate IR (Wilkin et al., 2004). Youth with obesity and IR are at increased risk of associated chronic conditions in adulthood, such as elevated blood pressure (BP),

* Corresponding author: Ruth C. Bindler, RNC, PhD.
E-mail address: bindler@wsu.edu (R.C. Bindler).

0882-5963/$ – see front matter © 2013 Elsevier Inc. All rights reserved.
http://dx.doi.org/10.1016/j.pedn.2012.03.022

cardiovascular disease (CVD), T2D, and several types of cancers (Adam et al., 2009; Biro & Wien, 2010; Li et al., 2009).

Despite the known relationships between IR and cardiometabolic factors, no study has yet examined the independent effects of these factors on a predictive model of IR among early adolescents. Such a predictive model would provide important information for health care providers to plan for evaluative assessments that will most reliably predict IR. Therefore, the purposes of this study among a group of early adolescents participating in the Teen Eating and Activity Mentoring in Schools (TEAMS) study were to describe the anthropometric and laboratory markers of the participants and to test the ability of these markers to predict risk of exhibiting IR.

The specific aims of this study were to

1. contrast prevalence of IR and other cardiometabolic risk factors in male and female adolescents;
2. contrast prevalence of IR and other cardiometabolic risk factors in adolescents according to weight status;
3. examine correlates of IR with anthropometric and laboratory markers among adolescents; and
4. determine if lipids/triglycerides, inflammatory markers, and weight status can reliably predict IR in adolescents.

Materials and Methods

Participants

Participants included all middle school students who volunteered to participate in a project called TEAMS. The TEAMS study was designed to improve health of participants at four schools through environmental changes in the nutrition policies of the school and individual interventions with participants. The research described herein reflects cross-sectional data analysis on the convenience sample recruited into TEAMS. Data for this study were collected at baseline and do not reflect any potential intervention effects. Students were recruited during open houses at the middle schools, during school-based barbeques for families, through school newsletters, and by school and study personnel in the first month of the student attendance in seventh grade. Students with mental or physical conditions that would limit their participation in study activities or those taking insulin or oral glycemic medications were excluded. Only one student of those recruited was excluded from the study based on exclusionary criteria.

Procedures

University and school district institutional review board approvals and signed parent permission/student assent were obtained. Students participated in assessments at their respective schools or at the university campus.

Fasting serum venipunctures were performed by licensed phlebotomists in the early morning, followed by a nutritious breakfast. Although some research demonstrates that non-fasting samples for lipids are similar to fasting samples (Langsted, Freiberg, & Nordestgaard, 2008), we chose to use fasting samples because all blood draws were to be done in early morning and because we were testing insulin and glucose, which are more accurate with fasting samples. Samples were transported within 1 hour to the laboratory for analysis. Total cholesterol, low-density lipoprotein–cholesterol (LDL-C), high-density lipoprotein–cholesterol (HDL-C), and triglycerides were measured by enzymatic method on Siemens Advia 2400 chemistry analyzer. High-sensitivity C-reactive protein (hsCRP) was measured by nephelometry on the Beckman-Coulter Immage 800. Glucose was tested using hexokinase method on the Siemens Advia 2400 C, and insulin was measured by chemiluminescent immunoassay on Immulite Analyzer.

The Homeostasis Model Assessment of Insulin Resistance (HOMA-IR) was chosen as the method for measuring IR in this study because it is recognized as a reliable test for IR, is a strong indicator of metabolic syndrome (MS) in youth, and is related to both longitudinal changes and adiposity (Conwell, Trost, Brown, & Batch, 2004; Gungor, Saad, Janosky, & Arslanian, 2004; Keskin, Kurtoglu, Kendrici, Atabek, & Yazici, 2005; Puder, Schindler, Zahner, & Kriemler, 2010; Sharma, Lustig, & Fleming, 2011; Yeckel et al., 2004). HOMA-IR was calculated as insulin (μU/ml) × glucose (mg/dl) / 405.0. Lower HOMA-IR scores indicate greater insulin sensitivity, whereas higher HOMA-IR scores reflect greater IR at the cellular level (Conwell et al., 2004; Gungor et al., 2004; Keskin et al., 2005; Lee et al., 2006; Yeckel et al., 2004).

Anthropometric measurement of students by trained personnel included height and weight. Height was measured on a standing stadiometer with shoes, hair ornaments, hats, jewelry, and braids removed. Participants were instructed to stand tall facing forward with feet together and heels, buttocks, shoulder blades, and back of head in contact with the vertical backboard. The upper measure of the stadiometer was aligned, and the participant stepped away. The height was measured and recorded in feet and inches with two decimal points as needed. Weight was measured on a Seca digital scale with shoes, coats, and other heavy clothing removed. The electronic display was positioned so it was visible only to the examiner and the person being weighed. Weight was recorded in pounds with two decimal points as needed. BMI was then calculated by dividing weight in pounds by height in inches squared, and multiplying by a conversion factor of 703 (Cole, Faith, Pietrobelli, & Heo, 2005). Exact BMI percentile for each adolescent was determined using the median (M), generalized coefficient of variation (S), and the power in the Box–Cox transformation (L) values for the patient's age in months and gender. This technique is referred to as the LMS method (http://www.cdc.gov/growthcharts/percentile_data_files.htm).

Systolic blood pressure (SBP) and diastolic blood pressure (DBP) were measured using the protocols of the

Appendix B

National Health and Nutrition Examination Survey (NHANES; CDC, 2005). Research participants sat quietly for 5 minutes. The largest cuff that would fit on the upper arm and leave room below for the head of the stethoscope was chosen, and the participant sat with the right arm supported on a table at heart level. The radial pulse was palpated while inflating the cuff, and the level at which the pulse was not palpable was noted; the cuff was then fully deflated. With the stethoscope on the brachial artery, the BP cuff was inflated to 20–30 mm Hg above the level of cessation of the radial pulse. The cuff was deflated 2 mm Hg per second noting the SBP and DBP. For two additional times, the participant sat quietly for 2 minutes, and the BP was measured again. As recommended by NHANES, the first BP measurement was not used in calculation; the remaining two SBP and DBP readings were averaged for use in the study. BP percentiles were reached using the National Heart, Lung and Blood Institute BP tables, which take into account the height percentile, gender, and age of participants (Falkner & Daniels, 2004; Pickering et al., 2005).

Statistical Analysis

Descriptive data were reported for each measure as the mean of all participants with standard deviation. Study outcome variables were assessed for normality using the Kolmogorov–Smirnov statistic and by examination of histograms and normal Q-Q plots. Mean differences by gender and by weight status were examined using independent samples *t* tests. Levene's test of equality of variance was performed to determine the appropriate *t* test for equality of means. Study authors recognized the skewed nature of HOMA-IR values among adolescents and accordingly log transformed HOMA-IR as the outcome variable of interest. Pearson correlation coefficients were used to examine relationships between study variables and IR as measured by the log transformation of HOMA-IR. Multicollinearity and multivariate outliers were assessed using collinearity diagnostics and Mahalanobis distances, respectively. A multiple regression model was developed using the log transformation of HOMA-IR as the dependent variable and other study variables as potential predictor variables.

Results

The first study aim was to contrast prevalence of cardiometabolic risk factors in male and female adolescents. A total of 150 early-adolescent participants were measured. Mean HOMA-IR was 2.93 ($SD = 2.44$). Gender differences in HOMA-IR were observed with female participants having higher HOMA-IR compared with males (Table 1). Mean age is 150.53 months or 12.54 years, with standard deviation of 4.17 months; the mean age of the females in the study was slightly lower than that of the males (12.50 vs. 12.60 years). The mean BMI, BMI percentile, and waist circumference of the female participants were higher than those of the males, whereas HDL-C was lower in females. There were no significant gender differences in hsCRP, triglycerides, total cholesterol, LDL-C, or BP.

The second study aim was to contrast the prevalence of IR and other risk factors in adolescents when considering weight status. Mean HOMA-IR also differed by weight status; we used BMI percentile to represent weight status differences (<95th percentile vs. ≥95th percentile; Table 2). Obese (BMI percentile ≥95th percentile) participants had mean HOMA-IR of 4.66 ($SD = 3.38$) compared with nonobese (BMI percentile < 95th percentile) individuals with mean HOMA-IR of 2.32 ($SD = 1.63$). Participants with obesity were younger than those who were not obese ($M =$

Table 1 Sample Characteristics by Gender

	All Participants ($N = 150$)		Males ($n = 64$)		Females ($n = 86$)		Gender Difference
	M	*SD*	*M*	*SD*	*M*	*SD*	*p*
*Age (months)	150.53	4.17	151.30	4.47	149.97	3.87	0.05
**BMI (kg/m^2)	22.32	5.12	21.05	4.30	23.27	5.48	0.006
*BMI percentile	70.83	26.61	65.83	26.85	74.56	25.97	0.05
*Waist circumference (cm)	77.49	13.20	74.77	12.21	79.53	13.62	0.03
*HOMA-IR	2.93	2.44	2.49	2.27	3.26	2.52	0.05
hsCRP (mg/dl)	1.21	1.99	1.29	2.42	1.15	1.62	0.69
Triglycerides (mg/dl)	93.73	44.16	86.48	39.10	99.12	47.08	0.08
Total cholesterol (mg/dl)	161.72	27.18	160.42	27.47	162.69	27.09	0.62
LDL-C (mg/dl)	96.84	23.61	95.97	23.68	97.49	23.69	0.70
HDL-C (mg/dl)	46.13	10.30	47.17	10.49	45.35	10.15	0.29
SBP (mm Hg)	104.84	10.86	105.83	10.44	104.12	11.17	0.36
DBP (mm Hg)	65.22	9.57	66.53	9.07	64.27	9.86	0.16

* $p \leq .05$.
** $p \leq .01$.

Table 2 Sample Characteristics by Weight Status (N = 150)

	BMI Percentile <95th (n = 111)		BMI Percentile ≥95th (n = 39)		Weight Status Difference
	M	*SD*	*M*	*SD*	*p*
**HOMA-IR	2.32	1.63	4.66	3.38	<0.001
**Waist circumference (cm)	71.69	7.66	94.13	11.55	<0.001
*hsCRP (mg/dl)	1.01	2.01	1.79	1.84	0.04
**Triglycerides (mg/dl)	87.24	42.82	112.18	43.21	0.002
Total cholesterol (mg/dl)	162.44	26.76	159.67	28.60	0.59
LDL-C (mg/dl)	96.91	22.84	96.64	26.01	0.95
**HDL-C (mg/dl)	48.09	9.97	40.54	9.24	<0.001
**SBP (mmHg)	101.77	10.11	113.00	8.36	<0.001
**DBP (mmHg)	63.38	9.85	70.13	6.74	<0.001

* $p \leq .05$.
** $p \leq .01$.

148.85 months vs. M = 151.13 months). HOMA-IR, waist circumference, hsCRP, triglycerides, SBP, and DBP were higher in youth with obesity, whereas HDL-C was significantly lower in youth with obesity.

Our third study aim was to examine correlates of IR among anthropometric and laboratory factors. Significant correlations were found, with higher HOMA-IR associated with elevated BMI, BMI percentile, waist circumference, hsCRP, triglycerides, and SBP; higher HOMA-IR was also associated with lower HDL-C (Table 3). There were nonsignificant correlations of HOMA-IR with total cholesterol, LDL-C, or DBP.

To answer the fourth study aim, regression modeling was conducted to determine whether factors (weight status, C-reactive protein [CRP], blood lipids, and BP) reliably predicted HOMA-IR. Several measures of obesity and central adiposity were considered as predictors of HOMA-IR, including BMI, BMI percentile, BMI *z*-scores, and waist circumference. Bivariate statistically significant independent variables of gender, age, multiple measures of adiposity, hsCRP, lipids, and BP did not increase explanatory power in this multivariate model and were excluded. The strongest predictive model included waist circumference (p = .002) and triglycerides ($p < .001$) as significant predictors of HOMA-IR, $F(2, 146) = 40.69$, $p < .001$. This model accounted for 35% of variance in HOMA-IR. Tolerance statistics and variance inflation factors (VIFs) were calculated and reviewed. The largest VIF of 1.136 indicated that multicollinearity was not demonstrated. A summary of the regression model is presented in Table 4.

Table 3 Bivariate Correlation With Log HOMA-IR (N = 150)

	r	*p*
Age (months)	−.088	0.29
**BMI (kg/m^2)	.539	<0.001
**BMI percentile	.353	<0.001
**Waist circumference (cm)	.560	<0.001
*hsCRP (mg/dl)	.172	0.04
**Triglycerides (mg/dl)	.363	<0.001
Total cholesterol (mg/dl)	−.119	0.15
LDL-C (mg/dl)	−.131	0.11
**HDL-C (mg/dl)	−.323	<0.001
**SBP	.215	0.01
DBP	.127	0.13

* $p \leq .05$.
** $p \leq .01$.

Discussion

This study of HOMA-IR among early adolescents in the TEAMS study described gender and weight status differences among participants, identified clinical variables associated with increased levels of HOMA-IR, and established a predictive model for HOMA-IR that would be useful in guiding clinicians who seek to prevent IR in youth. The model included a measure of central adiposity and levels of triglycerides as predictive variables of HOMA-IR.

Females in this study, although younger than males, were more likely to demonstrate obesity, with a mean BMI of 23.27 for females and 21.05 for males, and mean BMI percentile of 74.56 for females and 65.83 for males. Waist circumference, a measure of central adiposity, was also significantly higher in females than males (79.53 vs. 74.77 cm). There were more females than males in the study (86 vs.

Table 4 Multivariate Regression Model Predicting HOMA-IR (N = 150)

	B	*SE B*	*β*
Waist circumference	0.011	0.002	0.438
Triglycerides (mg/dl)	0.002	0.001	0.299

Note: R^2 = .35 ($p < .001$).

Appendix B

64), and it is possible that the study TEAMS appealed more to females who had higher BMI. Female HOMA-IR mean values were also higher than those of males by 0.77 points, a factor that could be associated with the greater number of females with higher BMI. Higher HOMA-IR scores in females were consistent with findings of some past studies (Lee et al., 2006; Moran et al., 1999) and differing from others which found females to be at a lower risk for MS than males (Weiss et al., 2004). Male participants in this study demonstrated lower levels of total cholesterol and LDL-C, and higher BP (both systolic and diastolic) as well as hsCRP, although none of these differences were significant. Triglycerides were lower in male adolescents than in female counterparts; males also had higher HDL-C than female test participants. This last finding is inconsistent with some other work, which finds lower HDL-C levels in adolescent males (Denney-Wilson, Hardy, Dobbins, Okely, & Baur, 2008), but may reflect the overall higher cardiometabolic risk status of females in the TEAMS study.

Higher BMI, BMI percentile, hsCRP, triglycerides, and SBP were associated with HOMA-IR, whereas low HDL-C was significantly correlated with increased HOMA-IR. Individuals with obesity had significantly higher levels of IR based on their HOMA-IR scores; this finding is consistent with other work (Kortoglu et al., 2010), but the levels in our study were strikingly increased. The participants with obesity also had significantly increased values of hsCRP and triglycerides, as well as both SBP and DBP.

Participants with obesity had significantly reduced levels of HDL-C compared with those of nonobese individuals in the study. Nonsignificant differences based on weight status were found in total cholesterol and LDL-C. The findings of this study were congruent with results among adolescents in previous research studies throughout the United States. Several cardiometabolic risks associated with obesity in this study reinforce prior work in this area. Being overweight is associated with dyslipidemia and high BP, both of which are risk factors for future CVD (Gilardini et al., 2006; Mertens & Van Gaal, 2000; Sinaiko, Donahue, Jacobs, & Prineas, 1999). Past studies have shown that obese adolescents are more likely to have higher levels of LDL-C and lower levels of HDL-C (Herder et al., 2007). Likewise, lower HDL-C levels are seen in those with obesity in the TEAMS study (Table 2); however, the levels of LDL-C in the test participants were not significantly elevated as predicted by previous studies.

CRP is associated with a pro-inflammatory state; central adiposity and higher levels of hsCRP have been found in adult patients with coronary artery disease and T2D (Gilardini et al., 2006; Lambert et al., 2004; Rubin et al., 2008; Weiss et al., 2004), and mild chronic levels of CRP are independent predictors of CVD in adults (Han et al., 2002). In recent studies, overweight children have had higher levels of CRP (Herder et al., 2007; Lambert et al., 2004), and relationships between CRP and BMI, as well as between CRP and fasting insulin values, have been noted (Lambert et al., 2004; Puder et al., 2010). It is still not well understood if CRP is a predictor or mediator of IR in adolescents (Lambert et al., 2004), and in some past research, elevated CRP was significantly related to obesity but not IR (Weiss et al., 2004). Park et al. (2009) noted that hsCRP is independently related to concurrent and future IR in young adults.

The identified factors that were independently associated with HOMA-IR—weight status, inflammatory marker hsCRP, some lipid levels, BP, age, and gender—were considered for a predictive model. Waist circumference, a measure of obesity and central adiposity, was chosen as the weight status variable. Although we found waist circumference to have the greatest explanatory power, similar results were reached with other measures of weight status. Rodriguez-Rodriguez, Palmeros-Exsome, Lopez-Sobaler, and Ortega (2010) also found waist circumference to be a strong predictor of IR. Our final parsimonious model indicated that waist circumference and triglyceride levels were independent factors associated with IR, and so other factors were eliminated from the model. When waist circumference and triglyceride levels were entered into a multivariate regression model to predict HOMA-IR, the overall model significantly predicted greater than 35% of the variance in HOMA-IR for adolescents in this study.

Limitations

There are some limitations of this study that could have affected the results, the first of which was a small sample size. The study was cross sectional, and future work that is longitudinal will be helpful to examine changes in HOMA-IR over time among adolescents. Because study participants volunteered to participate, it is not known if the sample of students that volunteered to participate had similar or different anthropometric, laboratory, or BP measurements when compared with students who did not volunteer to be included in the study. It would have been ideal to measure pubertal status of the children because puberty is associated with increased IR; girls usually enter puberty earlier, and our sample was at an age when some were prepubertal and others postpubertal (Nelson & Bremer, 2010). However, the school district would not allow Tanner pubertal staging. In addition, the population in the city where the research was conducted is not ethnically diverse; the majority of the study participants were of European American descent. Finally, within the participants, there was a bias toward overweight or obesity. Nearly one half of the individuals in the TEAMS research study were either overweight or obese. Therefore, this work is exploratory in nature and should be foundational to further research that can lead to increased generalizability among adolescent populations.

In the future, a longitudinal study with more individuals would help to identify the trends of IR and related factors in a larger population over time. Relationships among weight status, inflammatory markers, lipids, and IR at a young age

should be followed longitudinally to identify developmental variations and health outcomes. A weight reduction and healthy eating intervention plan should be contrasted with a control group to examine if reduced weight status, improved inflammatory markers, and improved lipid levels would have an impact on IR. Finally, targeting a more diverse and representative population would be needed to generalize the results to other adolescents.

Implications for Pediatric Nurses

Youth obesity is a major worldwide health crisis, and its effects can be viewed as a multifaceted problem with potential long-term health consequences. Its influence on IR and its link with lipids, BP, and other metabolic abnormalities (Juarez-Lopez et al., 2010) are particularly important and may help to elucidate the relationship of obesity with T2D and other chronic diseases. The novel findings of this study are that simple tests commonly administered in the office, hospital, school, or clinic setting (weight status and triglyceride level) can be predictive of the presence of the serious problem of IR.

Pediatric nurses should always measure weight and height and then calculate BMI and BMI percentile for youth in all settings, being alert for those children and adolescents outside of the recommended weight for height parameters. Several bodies, such as the United States Preventive Services Task Force (USPSTF), the American Academy of Pediatrics (AAP), the American Heart Association (AHA), the National Association of Pediatric Nurse Practitioners (NAPNAP), the CDC, and the American Medical Association (AMA), make recommendations for assessment, prevention, and treatment of obesity in children, and they all begin with emphasis on the importance of regular weight status and BMI measurement (Barlow and the Expert Committee, 2007; AHA, 2008; AMA, 2007; NAPNAP, 2009; USPSTF, 2010). For all youth, preventive interventions should be implemented. These "upstream" approaches include teaching about topics such as eating five fruits and vegetables daily, integrating family dinners several times weekly, decreasing fast-food dining and sugared beverage intake, limiting screen activities to no more than 2 hours per day, engaging in daily vigorous physical activity, and other approaches suggested by the cultural and contextual history of the family.

When children and adolescents have a BMI above the 85th percentile, and particularly above the 95th percentile, additional information should be considered. Waist circumference is a significant weight status measurement and should be evaluated with children displaying high BMI percentiles; additional data should include BP, dietary analysis, physical activity patterns, lipid panels, and glucose and insulin relationship.

Youth identified with risk factors for IR and cardiometabolic outcomes need a "downstream" approach with more intensive teaching and additional interventions to lower risk, measure progress toward outcomes, and continue monitoring of their health status. Interventions may include establishing a dietary plan, prescribed physical activity program, motivational interviewing, support group, and continued monitoring of health outcomes. These interventions generally involve an interprofessional team, so the pediatric nurse must communicate directly with other team members, such as a physician, exercise specialist, psychologist, and others. The pediatric nurse, a key participant due to understanding of the community, school and family influences, is often an effective team manager for the child or adolescent with obesity and concomitant risk of IR.

This study compared prevalence of IR and related cardiometabolic risk factors in male and female adolescents, and by weight status. It examined relationships among cardiometabolic risk factors and tested a predictive model for HOMA-IR. Results reinforced the importance of measuring weight and height, calculating BMI, and gathering further assessment data in youth at risk.

Acknowledgments

This project was supported by Agriculture and Food Initiative Grant 2007-55215-17909 from the USDA National Institute for Food and Agriculture.

References

Adam, T. C., Toledo-Corral, C., Lane, C. J., Weigensberg, M. J., Spruijt-Metz, D., Davies, J. N., et al. (2009). Insulin sensitivity as an independent predictor of fat mass gain in Hispanic adolescents. *Diabetes Care*, *32*, 2114–2115.

American Heart Association. (2008). Policy position statement on the prevention, assessment, diagnosis and treatment of child and adolescent obesity in the healthcare environment. Retrieved from http://www.heart.org/idc/groups/heart-public/@wcm/@adv/documents/downloadable/ucm_301721.pdf.

American Medical Association. (2007). Expert committee recommendations on the assessment, prevention and treatment of child and adolescent overweight and obesity. *Pediatrics*, *120*(Supp 4), S164–S192. Retrieved from http://www.ama-assn.org/ama/pub/category/11759.html.

Barlow, S. E. and the Expert Committee. (2007). Expert committee recommendations regarding the prevention, assessment, and treatment of child and adolescent overweight and obesity: Summary report. *Pediatrics*, *120*, S164–S192.

Biro, F. M., & Wien, M. (2010). Childhood obesity and adult morbidities. *American Journal of Clinical Nutrition*, *91*, 1499S–1505S.

Bitsori, M., Linardakis, M., Tabakaki, M., & Kafatos, A. (2009). Waist circumference as a screening tool for the identification of adolescents with the metabolic syndrome phenotype. *International Journal of Pediatric Obesity*, *4*, 325–331.

Centers for Disease Control and Prevention. (2005). *Documentation, codebook and frequencies.* National Health and Nutrition Examination Survey 2003–2004. Washington, DC: Author.

Centers for Disease Control and Prevention. (2010). Children and diabetes. Retrieved from http://www.cdc.gov/diabetes/projects/cda2.htm.

Cole, T. J., Faith, M. S., Pietrobelli, A., & Heo, M. (2005). What is the best measure of adiposity change in growing children: BMI, BMI%, BMI *z*-score or BMI centile? *European Journal of Clinical Nutrition*, *59*, 419–425.

Conwell, L. S., Trost, S. G., Brown, W. J., & Batch, J. A. (2004). Indexes of insulin resistance and secretion in obese children and adolescents. *Diabetes Care*, *27*, 314–319.

Cossio, S., Messiah, S. E., Garibay-Nieto, M., Lopez-Mitnik, G., Flores, P., Arheart, K. L., et al. (2009). How do different indices of obesity correlate with cardiometabolic disease risk factors in multiethnic youths? *Endocrine Practice*, *15*, 403–409.

Denney-Wilson, E., Hardy, L. L., Dobbins, T., Okely, A. D., & Baur, L. (2008). Body mass index, waist circumference, and chronic disease risk factors in Australian adolescents. *Archives of Pediatrics and Adolescent Medicine*, *162*, 566–573.

Falkner, B., & Daniels, S. R. (2004). Summary of the fourth report on the diagnosis, evaluation, and treatment of high blood pressure in children and adolescents. *Hypertension*, *44*, 387–388.

Gilardini, L., McTenan, P. G., Girola, A., da Silva, N. F., Alberti, L., Kumar, S., et al. (2006). Adiponectin is a candidate marker of metabolic syndrome in obese children and adolescents. *Atherosclerosis*, *189*, 401–407.

Gungor, N., Saad, R., Janosky, J., & Arslanian, S. (2004). Validation of surrogate estimates of insulin in children and adolescents. *Journal of Pediatrics*, *144*, 47–55.

Han, T. S., Sattar, N., Williams, K., Gonzalez-Villalpando, C., Lean, M. E., & Haffner, S. M. (2002). Prospective study of CRP in relation to the development of diabetes and MS in the Mexico City Diabetes Study. *Diabetes Care*, *25*, 2016–2021.

Herder, C., Schneitler, S., Rathmann, W., Haastert, B., Schneitler, K., Horst, W., et al. (2007). Low-grade inflammation, obesity, and insulin resistance in adolescents. *Journal of Clinical Endocrinology and Metabolism*, *92*, 4569–4574.

Juarez-Lopez, C., Klunder-Klunder, M., Medina-Bravo, P., Madrigal-Azcarate, A., Mass-Diaz, E., & Flores-Huerta, S. (2010). Insulin resistance and its association with the components of the metabolic syndrome among obese children and adolescents. *BMC Public Health*, *10*, 318.

Keskin, M., Kurtoglu, S., Kendrici, M., Atabek, M. E., & Yazici, C. (2005). Homeostasis model assessment is more reliable than the fasting glucose/insulin ratio and quantitative insulin sensitivity check index for assessing insulin resistance among obese children and adolescents. *Pediatrics*, *115*, 500–503.

Kim-Dorner, S. J., Deuster, P. A., Zeno, S. A., Remaley, A. T., & Poth, M. (2010). Should triglycerides and the triglycerides to high-density lipoprotein cholesterol ratio be used as surrogates for insulin resistance? *Metabolism*, *59*, 299–304.

Kortoglu, S., Hatipoglu, N., Mazicioglu, M., Dendirci, M., Keskin, M., & Kondolot, M. (2010). Insulin resistance in obese children and adolescents: HOMA-IR cut-off levels in the prepubertal and pubertal periods. *Journal of Clinical Research in Pediatric Endocrinology*, *2*, 100–106.

Lambert, M., Delvin, E. E., Paradis, G., O'Loughlin, J., Hanley, J. A., & Levy, E. (2004). C-reactive protein and features of the metabolic syndrome in a population-based sample of children and adolescents. *Clinical Chemistry*, *50*, 1762–1768.

Langsted, A., Freiberg, J. J., & Nordestgaard, B. G. (2008). Fasting and nonfasting lipid levels. *Circulation*, *118*, 2047–2056.

Lee, J. M., Okumura, M. J., Davis, M. M., Herman, W. H., & Gurney, J. G. (2006). Prevalence and determinants of insulin resistance among U.S. adolescents. *Diabetes Care*, *29*, 2427–2434.

Li, C., Ford, E. S., Huang, T. T., Sun, S. S., & Goodman, E. (2009). Patterns of change in cardiometabolic risk factors associated with the metabolic syndrome among children and adolescents: The Fels Longitudinal Study. *Journal of Pediatrics*, *155*(S5), e9–e16.

Liu, B. W., Lu, Q., Ma, C. M., Wang, S. Y., Lou, D. H., Lou, X. L., et al. (2009). Factors associated with insulin resistance and fasting plasma ghrelin levels in adolescents with obesity and family history of Type 2 diabetes. *Experimental and Clinical Endocrinology and Diabetes*, *117*, 600–604.

Mager, D. R., Ling, S., & Roberts, E. A. (2008). Anthropometric and metabolic characteristics in children with clinically diagnosed nonalcoholic fatty liver disease. *Paediatrics and Child Health*, *13*, 111–117.

Mertens, I. L., & Van Gaal, L. F. (2000). Overweight, obesity, and blood pressure: The effects of modest weight reduction. *Obesity Research*, *8*, 270–278.

Monzavi, R., Dreimane, D., Geffner, M., Braun, S., Conrad, B., Klier, M., et al. (2006). Improvement in risk factors for metabolic syndrome and insulin resistance in youth who are treated with lifestyle intervention. *Pediatrics*, *117*, 1111–1118.

Moran, A., Jacobs, D., Steinberger, J., Hong, C. P., Prineas, R., Luepker, R., et al. (1999). Insulin resistance during puberty: Results from clamp studies in 357 children. *Diabetes*, *48*, 2039–2044.

National Association of Pediatric Nurse Practitioners. (2009). Position statement on the identification and prevention of overweight and obesity in the pediatric population. *Journal of Pediatric Health Care*, *23*, 15A–16A.

National Diabetes Information Clearinghouse. (2008). Insulin resistance and pre-diabetes. Retrieved from http://diabetes.niddk.nih.gov/DM/pubs/insulinresistance/.

Nelson, R. A., & Bremer, A. A. (2010). Insulin resistance and metabolic syndrome in the pediatric population. *Metabolic Syndrome and Related Disorders*, *8*, 1–14.

Nur, M. M., Newman, I. M., & Siqueira, L. M. (2009). Glucose metabolism in overweight Hispanic adolescents with and without polycystic ovary syndrome. *Pediatrics*, *124*, e496–e502.

Ogden, C. L., Carroll, M. D., Curtin, L. R., McDowell, M. A., Tabak, C. J., & Flegal, K. M. (2006). Prevalence of overweight and obesity in the United States, 1999–2004. *JAMA: The Journal of the American Medical Association*, *295*, 1549–1555.

Park, K., Steffes, M., Lee, D. H., Himes, J. H., & Jacobs, D. R. (2009). Association of inflammation with worsening HOMA-insulin resistance. *Diabetologia*, *52*, 2337–2344.

Pickering, T. G., Hall, J. E., Appel, L. J., Falkner, B. E., Graves, J. W., Hill, M. N., et al. (2005). Recommendations for blood pressure measurement in humans and experimental animals: Part 1: Blood pressure measurement in humans: A statement from the Subcommittee of Professional and Public Education of the American Heart Association Council on High Blood Pressure Research. *Circulation*, *111*, 697–716.

Puder, J. J., Schindler, C., Zahner, L., & Kriemler, S. (2010). Adiposity, fitness and metabolic risk in children: A cross-sectional and longitudinal study. *International Journal of Pediatric Obesity*, *6*, e297–306.

Rodriguez-Rodriguez, E., Palmeros-Exsome, C., Lopez-Sobaler, A., & Ortega, R. M. (2010). Preliminary data on the association between waist circumference and insulin resistance in children without a previous diagnosis. *European Journal of Pediatrics*, *170*, 35–43.

Rubin, D. A., McMurray, R. G., Harrell, J. S., Hackney, A. C., Thorpe, D. E., & Haqq, A. M. (2008). The association between insulin resistance and cytokines in adolescents: The role of weight status and exercise. *Metabolism*, *57*, 683–690.

Shah, A. S., Dolan, L. M., Kimball, T. R., Gao, Z., Khoury, P. R., Daniels, S. R., et al. (2009). Influence of duration of diabetes, glycemic control, and traditional cardiovascular risk factors on early atherosclerotic vascular changes in adolescents and young adults with Type 2 diabetes mellitus. *Journal of Clinical Endocrinology and Metabolism*, *94*, 3740–3745.

Sharma, S., Lustig, R. H., & Fleming, S. E. (2011). Identifying metabolic syndrome in African American children using fasting HOMA-IR in place of glucose. *Preventing Chronic Disease*, *8*, A64.

Sinaiko, A., Donahue, R., Jacobs, D., & Prineas, R. (1999). Relation of weight and rate of increase in weight during childhood and adolescence to body size, BP, fasting insulin, and lipids in young adults: The

Minneapolis Children's Blood Pressure Study. *Circulation, 99,* 1471–1476.

United States Preventice Services Task Force. (2010). Screening for obesity in children and adolescents. *Pediatrics, 125,* 361–367. Retrieved from http://www.uspreventiveservicestaskforce.org/uspstf.uspschobes.htm

Weiss, R., Dziura, J., Burgert, T., Tamborlane, W., Taksali, S., Yeckel, C., et al. (2004). Obesity and the metabolic syndrome in children and adolescents. *New England Journal of Medicine, 350,* 2362–2374.

Wilkin, T. J., Voss, L. D., Metcalf, B. S., Mallam, K., Jeffery, A. N., Alba, S., et al. (2004). Metabolic risk in early childhood: The EarlyBird Study. *International Journal of Obesity, 28,* 564–569.

World Health Organization. (2011). Obesity and overweight. Retrieved from http://www.who.int/mediacentre/factsheets/fs311/en/index.html.

Yeckel, C. W., Weiss, R., Dziura, J., Taksali, S. E., Dufour, S., Burgert, T. S., et al. (2004). Validation of insulin sensitivity indices from oral glucose tolerance test parameters in obese children and adolescents. *Journal of Clinical Endocrinology and Metabolism, 89,* 1096–1101.

Appendix B

APPENDIX C

Knapp et al. Study

Applied Nursing Research 26 (2013) 51–57

Contents lists available at SciVerse ScienceDirect

Applied Nursing Research

journal homepage: www.elsevier.com/locate/apnr

Original Articles

The EPICS Family Bundle and its effects on stress and coping of families of critically Ill trauma patients

Sandra J. Knapp PhD, RN [a,*], Mary Lou Sole PhD, RN [b], Jacqueline Fowler Byers PhD, RN [c]

[a] University of Florida College of Nursing, PO Box 100187, Gainesville, FL 32606, USA
[b] UCF College of Nursing, PO Box 162210, Orlando, FL 32816, USA
[c] PO Box 162210, Orlando, FL 32826, USA

ARTICLE INFO

Article history:
Received 28 February 2012
Revised 5 November 2012
Accepted 7 November 2012

Keywords:
Critical care
Trauma
Families
Stress
Coping

ABSTRACT

Aim: The aim of this study was to evaluate impact of the EPICS Family Bundle on stress and coping.
Background: Critical care nurses frequently deal with family stress, but may be without knowledge and skills needed to assist families to cope.
Methods: A non-equivalent control group design was used, with a convenience sample of 84 family members of critically ill patients. During the control phase, participants completed tools measuring stress and coping. The intervention included use of the EPICS Family Bundle. After implementation, participants completed the same tools as those administered during the control phase. Outcomes were analyzed using independent-sample *t*-tests.
Results: The experimental group had a significantly higher coping score on two subscales; and although not statistically significant, it was also improved on an additional four.
Conclusion: After implementation of the intervention, families experienced improved coping. The study may have lacked sufficient power to detect all differences.

1. Introduction

Families of critically ill patients experience stress related to the hospitalization of their family members, and their ability to cope varies. Stress may result in behavioral changes, exhaustion, decreased amount or quality of sleep, poor eating habits, worsening of health problems, and post-traumatic stress disorder (Auerbach et al., 2005; Carter & Clark, 2005; McAdam & Puntillo, 2009; Van Horn & Tesh, 2000). Nurses play an important role in assisting families to manage stress and cope (Chui & Chan, 2007; Engstrom & Soderberg, 2007; Hickey & Lewandowski, 1988). However, this assistance varies greatly among nurses, making its delivery inconsistent.

While needs and stressors of families of the critically ill have been researched extensively (Auerbach et al., 2005; Burchfield, Hamilton, & Banks, 1982; Hweidi, 2007; Leske, 2000; Plowfield, 1999; Yang, 2008), no studies have been conducted to determine if a formal educational nursing program was effective in reducing family stress and promoting coping. One qualitative study researched the use of reflective practice interventions on families of pediatric patients, but the nurses were studied rather than the families (Peden-McAlpine, Tomlinson, Forneris, Genck, & Meiers, 2005). Other research indicated that involving family members in providing oral care to cardiovascular patients decreased family stress, but the intervention was family involvement, not nursing education (Silvernale, Williamson, & King, 2006). Recently, the designation of a family care specialist (FCS) was found to be helpful for families when care of their loved ones was being withdrawn (Kirchhoff, Palzkill, Kowalkowski, Mork, & Gretarsdottir, 2009). However, placement of the FCS, not effects of education, was the intervention studied. This study evaluated the effectiveness of a group of evidence-based principles, a "family bundle", to reduce stress and improve coping in families of critically ill trauma patients. These principles were based on effective actions of nurses when providing family care. The intervention was termed the EPICS Family Bundle and consisted of five principles: Evaluate, Plan, Involve, Communicate, and Support, to guide rather than dictate interventions. In this way, the bundle could be tailored to meet the needs of the individual family members and in varying situations.

The bundle is implemented by the nurse when the family member is first met. A quick assessment (evaluation) can indicate what the next steps should be and how interventions will be adapted to the individual. For example, at first introduction, the nurse may determine that the patient's wife probably has a limited education by the way she has difficulty reading provided documents (*evaluation*). A short interview could provide more information. It could be determined at that time what the education level is and how information is best provided. Knowing this, the nurse will include it

* Corresponding author. Tel.: +1 352 273 6319(Office), +1 352 260 2358(Home); fax: +1 352 273 6536.
E-mail addresses: sjknapp@ufl.edu (S.J. Knapp), Mary.Sole@ucf.edu (M.L. Sole), JacquieByers@gmail.com (J.F. Byers).

0897-1897/$ – see front matter © 2013 Elsevier Inc. All rights reserved.
http://dx.doi.org/10.1016/j.apnr.2012.11.002

in her *plans* for family care. It may have also been determined at initial assessment that the wife feels helpless but wants to do something. The nurse could *involve* her in care by having her perform simple tasks such as oral care or assisting with turning. *Communication* has already been addressed. *Support* would be provided based on what the wife needs.

The specific aim of this research study was to assess the effectiveness of an evidence-based intervention for critical care nurses to assist families of critically ill trauma patients in reducing their stress and improving coping skills. The objectives were to evaluate the EPICS Family Bundle, change unit culture to one more conducive to family care, and to provide improved care for family members.

2. Theoretical framework

The research study is based on Lazarus and Folkman's Transactional Model of Stress and Coping. Lazarus and Folkman view stress as a psychological reaction response and define it as a relationship between a person and the environment that is considered taxing by the person and endangers well-being, and coping consists of cognitive and behavioral efforts to manage stressors. The theory suggests that a stressor is perceived by a person on an individual basis that is related to perception of the environment, and coping is accomplished by adapting thoughts and actions according to how the person views the stressor. The reaction between person and environment is reciprocal and bidirectional—one is caused and affected by the other (Lazarus & Folkman, 1984).

According to Lazarus and Folkman (1984), the stressed person conducts first a primary and then a secondary appraisal. During primary appraisal, the person identifies the stressor. Once the stressor is identified, secondary appraisal occurs, and the individual evaluates what might and can be done. Both primary and secondary appraisal of the stressor facilitate coping.

In the critical care setting, the family and its members are stressed by the critical care experience. How the experience is appraised initially and secondarily determines how coping will occur, whether effectively or ineffectively. Nurses who are knowledgeable in working with families can help to strengthen family members' coping mechanisms. Therefore, by following Lazarus and Folkman's theory, it can be assumed nurses can make a difference by intervening at a point that will help families (both as individuals and as systems) make a secondary appraisal of their stressful situation that will facilitate effective coping. Fig. 1 illustrates this process.

3. Methods

3.1. Design

A quasi-experimental design, nonequivalent control group, pretest–posttest design was used to conduct the study.

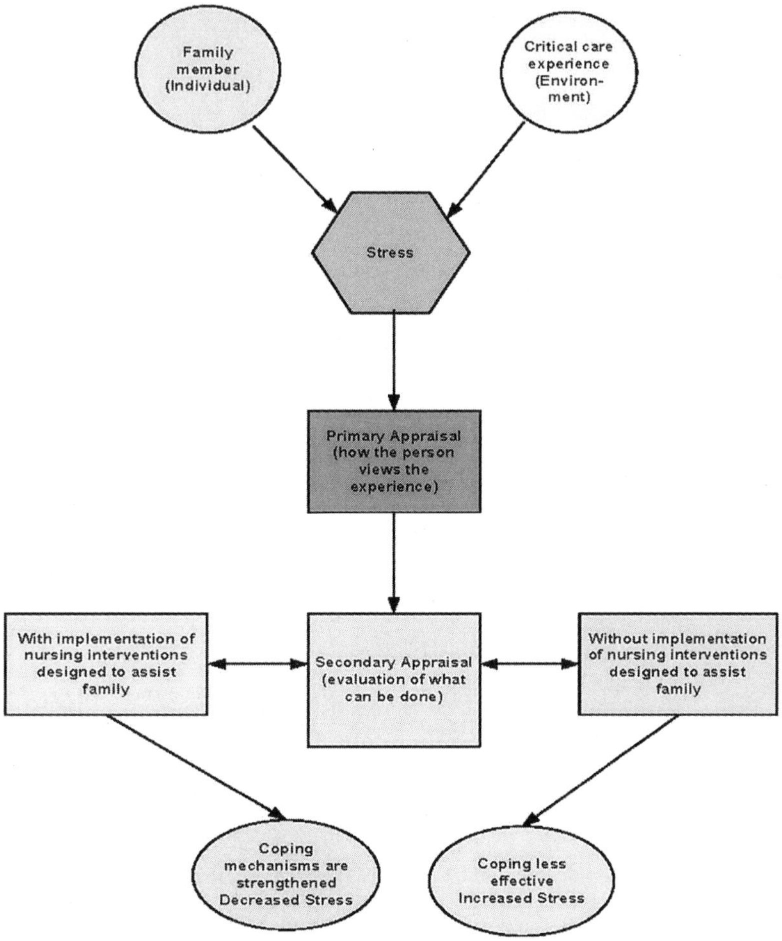

Fig. 1. Lazarus and Folkman's Transactional Cognitive Theory of Stress as applied to family members' critical care experience with and without assistive interventions by nursing.

S.J. Knapp et al. / Applied Nursing Research 26 (2013) 51–57 53

3.2. Ethical considerations

The study was approved by the institutional review boards (IRB) at the research site and the University of Central Florida. All participants signed an informed consent, and were issued a unique identification number to ensure confidentiality.

3.3. Sample

Participants were family members of critically ill trauma patients who had been admitted to the surgical intensive care unit (SICU) for at least 48 hours. Family members were at least 18 years old; spouse, parent, child, sibling, or significant other; and able to read and complete study tools in English. Participants were selected by convenience sampling, and no more than two family members per patient participated. The target sample size was 134 participants (67 in each group). Sample size estimates were based on an independent sample *t*-test assuming a medium effect size, alpha = .05, and power .80.

3.4. Setting

The study was conducted in the 30-bed SICU at a 617-bed tertiary university medical center in north central Florida with a level-1 trauma center. At the time, the SICU admitted patients with trauma, transplant, orthopedic, oncology, neurosurgery, and vascular surgery diagnoses (Marker, 2008). This study focused solely on the trauma population. An average of 28.5 trauma patients were admitted monthly to the SICU, and their average length of stay was 4.5 days (Ziglar, 2008).

3.5. Variables

The independent variable was implementation of the EPICS Family Bundle. Dependent variables were stress experienced by family members and their ability to cope.

3.6. Instruments

Instruments used to measure stress and coping were the State-Trait Anxiety Inventory (STAI) and the Ways of Coping Questionnaire (WAYS). Demographic data and the perception of needs being met were also collected.

3.7. Stress

The STAI has been used in many studies to measure the effects of an intervention on stress or anxiety in a variety of populations, including families of the critically ill. It is a self-reporting tool consisting of 40 statements: 20 related to state anxiety, and 20 related to trait anxiety with higher scores representing higher anxiety. A four-point Likert-type rating scale is used (Spielberger, 1983). The tool has been widely used in assessing stress and anxiety in the critical care setting and in conjunction with the Critical Care Family Needs Inventory (CCFNI) (Bormann, Smith, Shively, Dellefield, & Gifford, 2007; Chartier & Coutu-Wakulczyk, 1989; Chien, Chiu, Lam, & Ip, 2006; Delva, Vanoost, Bijttebier, Lauwers, & Wilmer, 2002; Kloos, 2004; LeBlanc & Bandiera, 2007; Soderstrom & Grimm, 2004; Spielberger, 1983).

Cronbach's alpha for the normative studies was consistently greater than .86, verifying internal consistency (Spielberger, 1983). In this study, the Cronbach's alpha was .92 for both state and trait anxiety. Test–retest reliability was assessed in the study population by administering the instruments twice on the same day to two participants. Agreement was 98% with both participants.

3.8. Coping

WAYS is a self-reporting tool that is widely used to assess coping. It consists of 66 items and uses a four-point Likert-type scale. Eight coping subscales are derived from 50 items on the tool. Internal consistency of the WAYS ranges 0.61 to 0.79. Possible scores range from 0 to 198, with higher scores representing more use of coping skills. The tool is recommended by the authors as useful for individual from high school through adult ages, so it is appropriate for this research study. It takes approximately 10 minutes to complete (Folkman & Lazarus, 1988).

In this study, data from the WAYS were evaluated in three ways: total score on the 66 items (WAYS 66), total score on the 50 items (WAYS 50), and scores on the subscales. Reliability statistics for these scores in this study were comparable to those reported by Folkman and Lazarus (1988).

3.9. EPICS intervention

The EPICS intervention the staff nurses' involved use of the EPICS Family Bundle when interacting with family members of critically ill trauma patients. Preparation for the intervention consisted of education with the staff nurses and identification of staff nurse champions to assist with implementation. The principal investigator (PI) provided ongoing follow-up throughout the eight-week study.

3.9.1. Education on the bundle

A program was developed to educate nurses on how to most effectively help their patients' families by using the EPICS Family Bundle. Five evidence-based concepts that are to be used when interacting with family members were emphasized: evaluate, plan, involve, communicate, and support. For the plan to be embraced and implemented by staff, nurses needed to change their customary practices in addition to receiving education, so preparation for the intervention also addressed changing the behavior and beliefs of the nurses.

The program was designed as a computer-based course that met state requirements for trauma-related continuing education (two contact hours). It was made available to all nurses. The course outlined the EPICS Family Bundle and included tactics that would help decrease stress and improve coping of family members. Related theoretical research and interventions found effective by researchers were included.

3.9.2. Pre-implementation strategies

Prior to initiating the educational program, the bundle was introduced to nurses by providing pens and flashlights that had the EPICS logo imprinted on them. The intention was to make the logo visible before the intervention, so an association could be made once education began. Once implementation began, the same logo with the

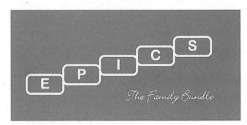

E P I C S
The Family Bundle

Fig. 2. EPICS logo.

addition of "The Family Bundle" was used throughout the program. The logo is illustrated with the addition in Fig. 2.

3.9.3. Pilot Testing

Two experts in family-centered critical care who were both doctorally prepared evaluated the content validity of the program. Three critical care nurses who worked in a different unit pilot tested the computer-based educational component of the program. Minor adjustments to the program were made after the pilot testing. All instruments and procedures were pilot-tested on a sample of five family members prior to initiating the study.

3.9.4. Introduction of the intervention

To launch the family-centered initiative, supplemental posters were placed throughout the SICU. Colorful flyers introducing key concepts were placed in various locations visible to staff, such as beside the central monitors and in the staff rest room. A one-page bulletin, "The Trauma Times", was posted in the nurses' lounge. Six weeks after the introduction of the Web-based education and related visual materials, four inservices were provided by the PI. All nurses were invited to participate, and they were provided with information and the opportunity for open discussion, communication, and an exchange of ideas.

3.9.5. Champions

The PI served as champion for the intervention, and key staff nurses who worked in the SICU on all shifts were selected as co-champions. Nurses were selected based on their experience and positions in the unit as preceptors, charge nurses, and their leadership and role modeling of family-centered care. Designation as co-champion was voluntary. Co-champions served as leaders and advisors to other staff members who were attempting to incorporate the EPICS Family Bundle into their nursing care. They acted as "sounding boards", offered advice, and acted as leaders. The PI met with the co-champions in group meetings early in the program and midway, and also individually throughout the 8 week program to provide guidance, support, and recommendations throughout the implementation, and to obtain feedback.

3.10. Data collection procedures

The study was conducted in three phases: pre-testing (control group), the intervention, and post-testing (intervention group).

3.10.1. Pre-testing

Pre-testing occurred prior to introduction of the intervention to gather data on the control group. Potential family member participants were identified by designated unit personnel. If they agreed to be contacted, the PI or designee discussed the study with them. Consent was obtained, and a packet with the research instruments (STAI, WAYS, and demographic tools) was given to participants. They were provided with a private area, such as a family conference room, to complete forms to maintain confidentiality. Most family members, however, preferred to remain at the bedside. A box was placed in a convenient area for survey responses to be deposited. Data were not analyzed until after study completion. Data were collected for 3 months from September to December, 2008.

3.10.2. Intervention

The intervention was implemented over an 8 week period.

3.10.3. Post-testing (intervention group)

Eight weeks after implementation of the intervention, eligible family members were recruited to participate in the study following the same procedures as the pre-test phase. Data were collected for three months, from January to April, 2009.

3.11. Data analysis

The STAI and WAYS were scored according to authors' instructions. Data were entered into Statistical Package for the Social Sciences v. 14 (Chicago, IL) for analysis (Statistical Package for the Social Sciences, 2005). Demographic characteristics were described using frequencies and descriptive statistics. Characteristics of the two groups of family members were tested to assess equivalence using chi-square statistics or independent *t*-test. Data from the STAI and WAYS were analyzed using one-tailed tests, with a priori alpha level set at .05. *T*-tests were conducted to analyze continuous data, and chi-square tests were run to analyze categorical data. All data were screened for outliers. Assumptions related to statistical tests were assessed.

3.12. Results

3.12.1. Sample characteristics

Data were collected on 39 family members in the control group and 45 in the intervention group. Average age for participants and patients ranged from 46 to 50; and the duration of patient hospitalization at the time of the study was 4.5 days. Demographic data for the sample are shown in Table 1. No differences ($p>.05$) were noted in characteristics of participants in the control and intervention groups: age, gender, relationship to patient, ethnicity, and race. Likewise, no differences were noted in the patients' characteristics of age and duration of hospitalization in the SICU.

3.13. Effects of EPICS on stress and coping

It was not expected that trait anxiety would be affected, but it was measured to determine participants' baseline stress. However, no significant differences either state or trait anxiety, both indirect measures of stress, were noted between groups ($p>.05$). No significant differences were noted for coping with the total WAYS (both WAYS 66

Table 1
Demographic data for family member participants.

Demographics	Control ($n=39$)	Experimental ($n=45$)	*p* value
Relationship to patient			.970[a]
Husband/wife	10	13	
Parent	11	13	
Child	10	11	
Brother/sister	6	6	
Significant other/partner	3	2	
Gender			.375[a]
Male	9	14	
Female	30	30	
Missing	0	1	
Ethnicity			.766[a]
Hispanic or Latino	2	3	
Not Hispanic or Latino	37	42	
Race			.316[a]
White	36	38	
Black or African American	1	5	
Other	2	2	
Participant (family member) age			.632[b]
Mean	45.92	47.38	
Range	22–77	19–79	
Patient age			.503[b]
Mean	47.87	50.27	
Range	19–83	21–90	
Patient days in the SICU			.633[b]
Mean	5.18	4.89	
Range	3–16	2–16	

[a] Chi square test.
[b] Independent samples *t*-test.

and 50) score between groups ($p > .05$). Analyzing each WAYS coping factor, it was found that those in the experimental group had significantly *higher* scores on the Distancing and Accepting Responsibility WAYS subsets ($p = .02$ and .006 respectively). Although not statistically significant, higher scores were also noted in the experimental group for confrontive coping, self-controlling, planful problem solving, and positive reappraisal subsets. Table 2 provides more detail on the effects of the EPICS intervention on coping.

4. Discussion

4.1. Stress

No differences in family stress were noted after the EPICS Family Bundle was initiated. It was hoped that implementation of the bundle would assist family members in decision-making, resulting in less state anxiety ("right now, at this moment") (Spielberger, 1983). Due to the unexpected, intense, and critical nature associated with traumatic injury, it may be difficult to impact the stress response solely through the implementation of a family bundle. Also, it is possible that the study was underpowered to attain a true assessment of the impact of the intervention.

4.2. Coping

Distancing and *accepting responsibility* subsets of coping were statistically significant between the two groups. Higher scores were found in the experimental group, indicating improved coping in these two subsets after implementation of the bundle.

Table 2
Coping, total scores and subsets.

Subset	Mean	Standard deviation	Min–Max	T	p (one-tailed)
Confrontive coping				−1.374	.087
Control	4.74	3.13	0–12		
Experimental	5.78	3.69	0–16		
Distancing				−2.030	.023
Control	4.00	2.51	0–12		
Experimental	5.27	3.11	0–14		
Self-controlling				−1.459	.075
Control	7.69	4.12	0–15		
Experimental	8.87	3.09	2–16		
Seeking social support				.364	.359
Control	10.49	3.94	2–18		
Experimental	10.18	3.83	0–17		
Accepting responsibility				−2.578	.006
Control	1.59	2.23	0–8		
Experimental	3.11	3.15	0–12		
Escape-avoidance				.166	.435
Control	8.62	4.54	0–20		
Experimental	8.44	4.85	0–20		
Planful problem solving				−.115	.454
Control	8.19	3.90	1–16		
Experimental	8.29	3.82	0–17		
Positive reappraisal				−.552	.291
Control	9.72	4.63	3–21		
Experimental	10.31	5.14	0–20		
Total (50)				−1.169	.123
Control	55.04	18.29	20–100		
Experimental	60.24	21.98	25–115		
Total (66)				−1.287	.101
Control	75.23	23.64	30–132		
Experimental	82.33	26.50	35–146		

Distancing is defined as "cognitive efforts to detach oneself and to minimize the significance of the situation" (Folkman & Lazarus, 1988, p. 7). The obvious demonstration would be simply not being present, which would be a negative response. Some family members, however, use other tactics in a positive way that mirror distancing, such as staying busy or distancing themselves emotionally rather than physically. For example, if family members receive the information they need, it is possible that this helps them with distancing by allowing their focus to become more on the health care plan of the patient than the injury or illness itself.

Family members who are well informed (which involves using the five components of the EPICS Family Bundle) adjust better than those who are not provided with information, because the need to be informed is met (Åstedt-Kurki, Paavilainen, Tammentie, & Paunonen-Ilmonen, 2001; Soderstrom, Saveman, & Benzein, 2006). In one study, distancing was found to occur more frequently when levels of distress were lower (Dunkel-Schetter, Feinstein, Taylor, & Falke, 1999). It is possible that due to the implementation of the bundle, family members were less distressed and therefore used distancing as a coping mechanism. Those who distance themselves in a negative way are not present to receive the information, and finding a way to update them could alleviate some family anxiety and promote coping.

The nurse who uses the EPICS Family Bundle will be able to determine through *evaluation* if distancing is occurring, and whether it is negative or positive. Interventions can be *planned* accordingly. *Involvement* will be tailored according to distancing style. *Communication* of information such as changes in patient condition will be of particular importance to those who distance themselves negatively, since their presence may not be very frequent. Less frequent visits and minimal participation could mean the family member needs additional emotional *support*, and the nurse would be able to recognize this.

Accepting responsibility is defined as "acknowledges one's own role in the problem with a concomitant theme of trying to put things right" (Folkman & Lazarus, 1988, p. 7).Family members want information and to be involved in patient care (Chan & Twinn, 2007; Davidson, Daly, Agan, Brady, & Higgins, 2010; Jacobowski, Girard, Mulder, & Ely, 2010; Molter, 1979). By providing information while involving them in care of their loved ones, nurses promote family members as having specific roles rather than simply being bystander s (Farvis, 2002). Family members experience a sense of control and assume responsibility when they receive continuous information (Lefebvre, Pelchat, Swaine, Gélinas, & Levert, 2005; Soderstrom et al., 2006). Involvement in care has been identified as a family need (Leon & Knapp, 2008; Silvernale et al., 2006).

It is therefore reasonable to surmise that the EPICS Family Bundle, which includes communication and involvement, would have a significant impact on accepting responsibility. By *evaluating*, the nurse can determine how involved the family member wants to be, and patient and family care can be *planned* accordingly. The family member who uses this coping mechanism will likely want to be a part of patient care, so *involvement* can be included in the plan. *Communication* is very important to these family members, and the nurse can facilitate it. *Support* could be providing additional information to meet the needs of the inquisitive person, or possibly a referral to a support group.

Although not statistically significant, means were higher for the experimental group in both WAYS Total 50 and WAYS Total 66. A trend of improvement in coping skills was evident for the experimental group for all coping subsets except seeking social support and escape/avoidance. The small sample size may be one reason for the non-significant findings.

4.3. Limitations

It was not possible to achieve the desired sample size in the allocated time period for the study. Reasons included difficulty

recruiting subjects in the beginning of the study, and a lower than usual number of patients admitted to the unit during part of the study. The data collection period was not extended during either pre- or post-testing to avoid introducing extraneous variables that might influence findings.

It was planned that the intranet educational program would be mandatory for all staff members; however, management designated the program as optional. The program was completed by 52 of 120 (43%) staff members in the SICU. The intranet program contained the theoretical foundation of the EPICS Family Bundle. In-services, one-on-one training, posters, bulletins, and other educational items were intended to supplement the intranet program. Some of the strength of the intervention may have been lost by not having all staff members complete the educational program. Offering the program in several ways, such as booklet form, oral presentation, or intranet, may have been more beneficial. Despite having less than half of the staff participate in the educational initiatives, the addition of co-champions was a way to increase the momentum of implementation of the EPICS Family Bundle.

Several nurses did not fully support the intervention, and they may have influenced others. When approached individually by the researcher or co-champions, many nurses would speak of their use of the EPICS Family Bundle positively; but when approached as a group to discuss implementation of the bundle, none participated in the discussions. A tool to determine participating nurses' knowledge and perception may have helped in determining effectiveness of the bundle. However, those who did comment privately about the bundle had positive things to say, such as, "It really helped me a lot" and "I like it".

Education alone is not adequate for promoting a change within a nursing unit. Although five concepts adopted by organizations with successful culture changes were used as a part of the intervention, 8 weeks was likely not enough time for an actual culture change to occur (Knapp, 2006). Organizational culture changes are complex, take time, and require leadership (Kotter & Heskett, 1992). A number of the SICU nurses have worked on the unit for over 10 years, making culture change more difficult.

Ideally, a control group and intervention group are tested at the same time. If this had been possible, the effect may have been greater. However, it was impractical to implement a true experimental design. Such a design would have necessitated managing the patient population, dividing them into two groups (control and intervention), and then having two groups of nurses (one group educated on the EPICS Family Bundle and the other providing "usual family care"). This would have necessitated the involvement of nurse management, and even with this collaboration, the logistics of creating and maintaining this division of groups would have been extremely difficult if not impossible. Contamination across groups would also have been likely.

5. Implications for research and practice

Extensive research has been conducted on needs of families of the critically ill, but less research exists on stress and coping of these families. This study provided valuable information on strategies to introduce family-centered interventions. A firm foundation of information on how to decrease stress, and improve coping skills of families has been laid through this study, and it is anticipated it will promote evidence-based practice in the critical care setting. This foundation can also be expanded to other areas, such as emergency, rehabilitative services, or cardiovascular intensive care.

The EPICS Family Bundle could be used in a number of settings. For example, the end of life of a loved one is especially difficult for family members to manage in any setting. The bundle can be used to assist families who have loved ones at the end of life by giving the bedside nurse the structure needed to ensure families are evaluated, included in planning care, involved in the care of their dying loved ones, and supported. It can be also used in conjunction with family presence during resuscitation or invasive procedures. Many nurses are reluctant to embrace these practices because of the stress, possible negative effects on the performance of the team, and possible interference with procedures because the family requires attention (Demir, 2008; Kuzin et al., 2007; Meyers et al., 2004). By using the EPICS Family Bundle, structure is laid for the nurse to ensure the best care is provided for families in a way that is most efficient. Hospitals that incorporate shared governance should welcome a structured plan that can involve all staff in its efforts to promote family-centered care. Staff involvement coupled with managerial support should facilitate introduction, acceptance, and use of the EPICS Family Bundle.

5.1. Summary

This study evaluated whether or not the EPICS intervention would decrease stress and improve coping skills of families of critically ill trauma patients. Family coping on two subsets—distancing and accepting responsibility—was significantly improved after implementation of the EPICS Family Bundle. A more significant impact can be obtained in future expansions of this study by increasing sample size and power, strengthening the educational program, culture change approach and intervention, and allowing more time for the change to occur. It is hoped future interventions will bring about favorable changes for nurses and families of the critically ill.

Callouts

- Nurses play an important role in assisting families to manage stress and cope with the stressors; however, many critical care nurses may not know how to provide the needed assistance.
- Critical care nurses were educated on the EPICS Family Bundle, which was composed of five evidence-based principles that can guide the nurse in assisting families. Groups of families were evaluated for stress and coping before and after the intervention to determine the effectiveness of the intervention.
- No significant differences either state or trait anxiety, both indirect measures of stress, were noted between groups ($p > .05$).
- Family members in the experimental group (tested after the intervention) had significantly higher scores on the coping subsets distancing and accepting responsibility ($p = .02$ and .006).
- All other coping subsets except two showed improvement, but results were not statistically significant.
- It can be concluded that the EPICS Family Bundle does help nurses to assist families improve their coping skills, but more studies are needed.

References

Åstedt-Kurki, P., Paavilainen, E., Tammentie, T., & Paunonen-Ilmonen, M. (2001). Interaction between adult patients' family members and nursing staff on a hospital ward. *Scandinavian Journal of Caring Sciences*, *15*(2), 142–150.

Auerbach, S., Kiesler, D., Wartella, J., Rausch, S., Ward, K., & Ivatury, R. (2005). Optimism, satisfaction with needs met, interpersonal perceptions of the healthcare team, and emotional distress in patients' family members during critical care hospitalization. *American Journal of Critical Care*, *14*(3), 202–210.

Bormann, J. E., Smith, T. L., Shively, M., Dellefield, M. E., & Gifford, A. L. (2007). Quality toolbox. Self-monitoring of a stress reduction technique using wrist-worn counters. *Journal for Healthcare Quality: Promoting Excellence in Healthcare*, *29*(1), 45–52.

Burchfield, S. R., Hamilton, K. L., & Banks, K. L. (1982). Affiliative needs, interpersonal stress and symptomatology. *Journal of Human Stress*, *8*(1), 5–9.

Carter PA, & Clark AP. Assessing and treating sleep problems in family caregivers of intensive care unit patients. *Crit Care Nurse*, *25*(1)(2005), 16, 18–23; quiz 24–15.

Chan, K. -S., & Twinn, S. (2007). An analysis of the stressors and coping strategies of Chinese adults with a partner admitted to an intensive care unit in Hong Kong: An exploratory study. *Journal of Clinical Nursing*, *16*(1), 185–193.

Chartier, L., & Coutu-Wakulczyk, G. (1989). Families in ICU: Their needs and anxiety level. *Intensive Care Nursing*, *5*(1), 11–18.

Chien, W. -T., Chiu, Y. L., Lam, L. -W., & Ip, W. -Y. (2006). Effects of a needs-based education programme for family carers with a relative in an intensive care unit: A quasi-experimental study. *International Journal of Nursing Studies*, *43*(1), 39–50.

Appendix C

Chui, W. Y., & Chan, S. W. (2007). Stress and coping of Hong Kong Chinese family members during a critical illness. *Journal of Clinical Nursing*, *16*(2), 372–381.
Davidson, J. E., Daly, B. J., Agan, D., Brady, N. R., & Higgins, P. A. (2010). Facilitated sense making: A feasibility study for the provision of a family support program in the intensive care unit. *Critical Care Nursing Quarterly*, *33*(2), 177–189.
Delva, D., Vanoost, S., Bijttebier, P., Lauwers, P., & Wilmer, A. (2002). Needs and feelings of anxiety of relatives of patients hospitalized in intensive care units: Implications for social work. *Social Work in Health Care*, *35*(4), 33.
Demir, F. (2008). Presence of patients' families during cardiopulmonary resuscitation: Physicians' and nurses' opinions. *Journal of Advanced Nursing*, *63*(4), 409–416.
Engstrom, A., & Soderberg, S. (2007). Close relatives in intensive care from the perspective of critical care nurses. *Journal of Clinical Nursing*, *16*(9), 1651–1659.
Farvis, M. (2002). Clinical update. The family: An important nursing resource for holistic client care. *Australian Nursing Journal*, *10*(5), 17–19.
Folkman, S., & Lazarus, R. (1988). Ways of coping questionnaire sampler set. Menlo Park, CA: Consulting Psychologists Press Inc.
Hickey, M., & Lewandowski, L. (1988). Critical care nurses' role with families: A descriptive study. *Heart & Lung*, *17*(6 Pt 1), 670–676.
Hweidi, I. M. (2007). Jordanian patient's perception of stressors in critical care units: A questionaire survey. *International Journal of Nursing Studies*, *44*(2), 227–235.
Jacobowski, N. L., Girard, T. D., Mulder, J. A., & Ely, E. W. (2010). Communication in critical care: Family rounds in the intensive care unit. *American Journal of Critical Care*, *19*(5), 421–430, http://dx.doi.org/10.4037/ajcc2010656.
Kirchhoff, K., Palzkill, J., Kowalkowski, J., Mork, A., & Gretarsdottir, E. (2009). Preparing families of intensive care patients for withdrawal of life support: A pilot study, CE articla. *NTI News*, 9–12.
Kloos, J. A. (2004). Effect of family-maintained progress journal on families of critically ill patients. Ph.D., Case Western Reserve University (Health Sciences). Retrieved from. , http://ucfproxy.fcla.edu/login?URL=http://search.ebscohost.com/login.aspx?direct=true&db=rzh&AN=2005109761&site=ehost-live
Knapp, S. (2006). *Changing the tides: Using organizational culture change methods to revolutionize attitudes about families in an ICU. Systematic review.* Orlando, FL: University of Central Florida.
Kotter, J., & Heskett, J. (1992). *Corporate culture and performance.* New York: The Free Press.
Kuzin, J. K., Yborra, J. G., Taylor, M. D., Chang, A. C., Altman, C. A., Whitney, G. M., et al. (2007). Family-member presence during interventions in the intensive care unit: Perceptions of pediatric cardiac intensive care providers. *Pediatrics*, *120*(4), e895–e901, http://dx.doi.org/10.1542/peds.2006-2943.
Lazarus, R., & Folkman, S. (1984). *Stress, Appraisal, and Coping.* New York, NY: Springer Publishing Company.
LeBlanc, V. R., & Bandiera, G. W. (2007). The effects of examination stress on the performance of emergency medicine residents. *Medical Education*, *41*(6), 556–564.
Lefebvre, H., Pelchat, D., Swaine, B., Gélinas, I., & Levert, M. J. (2005). The experiences of individuals with a traumatic brain injury, families, physicians and health professionals regarding care provided throughout the continuum. *Brain Injury*, *19*(8), 585–597.
Leon, A., & Knapp, S. (2008). Involving family systems in critical care nursing: Challenges and opportunities. *Dimensions of Critical Care Nursing*, *27*(6), 255–262.
Leske, J. S. (2000). Family stresses, strengths, and outcomes after critical injury. *Critical Care Nursing Clinics of North America*, *12*(2), 237–244.
Marker, P. (2008). [Nurse Manager, Shands at U.F. SICU].
McAdam, J. L., & Puntillo, K. (2009). Symptoms experienced by family members of patients in intensive care units. *American Journal of Critical Care*, *18*(3), 200–209, http://dx.doi.org/10.4037/ajcc2009252.
Meyers, T. A., Eichhorn, D. J., Guzzetta, C. E., Clark, A. P., Klein, J. D., & Taliaferro, E. (2004). Family presence during invasive procedures and resuscitation: The experience of family members, nurses, and physicians... reprinted with permission from the American Journal of Nursing, 2000;100(2):32–42. *Topics in Emergency Medicine*, *26*(1), 61–73.
Molter, N. (1979). Needs of relatives of critically ill patients: A descriptive study. *Heart & Lung*, *8*, 332–339.
Peden-McAlpine, C., Tomlinson, P., Forneris, S., Genck, G., & Meiers, S. (2005). Evaluation of a reflective practice intervention to enhance family care. *Journal of Advanced Nursing*, *49*(5), 494–501.
Plowfield, L. A. (1999). Living a nightmare: Family experiences of waiting following neurological crisis. *The Journal of Neuroscience Nursing*, *31*(4), 231–238.
Silvernale, M., Williamson, M., & King, C. (2006). Family involvement with personal care in long-term cardiothoracic surgical patients in the intensive care unit. *American Journal of Critical Care*, *15*(3), 339.
Soderstrom, I. M., Saveman, B. I., & Benzein, E. (2006). Interactions between family members and staff in intensive care units—An observation and interview study. *International Journal of Nursing Studies*, *43*(6), 707–716.
Soderstrom, M., & Grimm, P. (2004). Measuring anxiety. In M. Frank-Stromberg, & S. Olsen (Eds.), *Instruments for clinical health-care research* (3rd ed.). . Sudbury, MA: Jones and Bartlett Publishers, Inc.
Spielberger, C. (1983). State-Trait Anxiety Inventory for adults sampler set: Manual, test booklet and scoring key. Menlo Park, CA: Mind Garden, Inc.
Statistical Package for the Social Sciences. (2005). SPSS for Windows Graduate Student Version (Version 14.0.0).
Van Horn, E., & Tesh, A. (2000). The effect of critical care hospitalization on family members: Stress and responses. *Dimensions of Critical Care Nursing*, *19*(4), 40–49.
Yang, S. (2008). A mixed methods study on the needs of Korean families in the intensive care unit. *The Australian Journal of Advanced Nursing*, *25*(4), 79–86.
Ziglar, M. (2008). All patients who have been discharged from the date of 7/1/2006 to 6/30/2007. In K. blinded_3 (Ed.), *Excel* (pp. 1–2). Gainesville, FL: Shands Teaching Hospital, Trauma Center.

Notes

Notes

1 F ab C
2 Eb Ab C
3 3 EB G Bb
4 1 F ab C
2 Eb Ab C
Eb G Bb
Eb G bb
F Ab C
Eb Ab C
Eb G Bb
F Ab C
Eb Ab C
Eb G Bb
Eb G bb
F Ab C
Eb G bb
Eb G bb
F Ab C

ELSEVIER
SAUNDERS
3251 Riverport Lane
Maryland Heights, Missouri 63043

Study Guide for Understanding Nursing Research:
Building an Evidence-Based Practice, Sixth edition

ISBN: 978-1-4557-7253-7

Notice

Knowledge and best practice in this field are constantly changing. As new research and experience broaden our understanding, changes in research methods, professional practices, or medical treatment may become necessary.

Practitioners and researchers must always rely on their own experience and knowledge in evaluating and using any information, methods, compounds, or experiments described herein. In using such information or methods they should be mindful of their own safety and the safety of others, including parties for whom they have a professional responsibility.

With respect to any drug or pharmaceutical products identified, readers are advised to check the most current information provided (i) on procedures featured or (ii) by the manufacturer of each product to be administered, to verify the recommended dose or formula, the method and duration of administration, and contraindications. It is the responsibility of practitioners, relying on their own experience and knowledge of their patients, to make diagnoses, to determine dosages and the best treatment for each individual patient, and to take all appropriate safety precautions.

To the fullest extent of the law, neither the Publisher nor the authors, contributors, or editors, assume any liability for any injury and/or damage to persons or property as a matter of products liability, negligence or otherwise, or from any use or operation of any methods, products, instructions, or ideas contained in the material herein.

Executive Content Strategist: Lee Henderson
Associate Content Development Specialist: Courtney Daniels
Senior Project Manager: Divya Krish
Production Services Manager: Hema Rajendrababu

Printed in the United States of America

Last digit is the print number: 9 8 7 6 5 4 3 2

Study Guide for Understanding Nursing Research

Building an Evidence-Based Practice

Sixth Edition

Susan K. Grove, Jennifer R. Gray, and Nancy Burns

Study Guide prepared by

Susan K. Grove, PhD, RN, ANP-BC, GNP-BC

Professor Emerita
College of Nursing
The University of Texas at Arlington
Adult Nurse Practitioner, Family Practice Irving, Texas
Arlington, Texas

Jennifer Gray, RN, PhD, FAAN

Professor
Associate Dean and Department Chair
Department of Nursing Administration, Education, and Research Programs
College of Nursing
The University of Texas at Arlington
Arlington, Texas

ELSEVIER
SAUNDERS